Physiology of Human Reproduction

Physiology of Human Reproduction

Notes for Students

George Osol, PhD

Professor Emeritus
Department of Obstetrics, Gynecology and
Reproductive Sciences
University of Vermont Larner College of Medicine
Burlington, VT, USA

WILEY Blackwell

This edition first published 2021
© 2021 John Wiley & Sons Ltd

The right of George Osol to be identified as the author of this work has been asserted in accordance with law.

Registered Offices
John Wiley & Sons, Inc., 111 River Street, Hoboken, NJ 07030, USA
John Wiley & Sons Ltd, The Atrium, Southern Gate, Chichester, West Sussex, PO19 8SQ, UK

Editorial Office
9600 Garsington Road, Oxford, OX4 2DQ, UK

For details of our global editorial offices, customer services, and more information about Wiley products visit us at www.wiley.com.

Wiley also publishes its books in a variety of electronic formats and by print-on-demand. Some content that appears in standard print versions of this book may not be available in other formats.

Library of Congress Cataloging-in-Publication Data

Names: Osol, George, author.
Title: Physiology of human reproduction : notes for students / George Osol.
Description: Hoboken, NJ : Wiley-Blackwell, 2021. | Includes index.
Identifiers: LCCN 2020026467 (print) | LCCN 2020026468 (ebook) | ISBN 9781119609582 (paperback) | ISBN 9781119609605 (Adobe PDF) | ISBN 9781119609575 (epub)
Subjects: MESH: Reproduction–physiology | Study Guide
Classification: LCC QP251 (print) | LCC QP251 (ebook) | NLM WQ 200.1 | DDC 612.6–dc23
LC record available at https://lccn.loc.gov/2020026467
LC ebook record available at https://lccn.loc.gov/2020026468

Cover Design: Wiley
Cover Image: © Chad Baker/Getty Images

Set in 11.5/13.5 pt STIX Two Text by SPi Global, Pondicherry, India
Printed and bound by CPI Group (UK) Ltd, Croydon, CR0 4YY

10 9 8 7 6 5 4 3 2 1

Contents

Acknowledgement

I would like to thank Wiley, particularly James Watson, Anne Hunt, and D. Vincent Rajan for their editorial assistance and guidance with the publication and copyediting process, and my family for their patience and support.

Key Concepts and Terms

Chapter 1: The Adult Male

1. Three basic requirements for male fertility
2. GnRH
3. LH and FSH
4. Pulsatile release
5. First vs. second messengers
6. Leydig cells
7. Action of LH
8. Testosterone
9. Sertoli cells
10. Three main types of sex steroids
11. Aromatization
12. Conversion of testosterone into estrogen
13. Action of FSH
14. Inhibin
15. Sertoli cell functions
16. The blood-testis barrier
17. Spatial relationships in males vs. females
18. Diverse actions of testosterone
19. Actions of testosterone *in utero*
20. Sexual differentiation
21. Androgens during puberty
22. DHT
23. 5α-reductase

Chapter 2: The Nonpregnant Adult Female

Introduction

Expediency of communication, instant access, and a vast database to surf and learn from are undeniable benefits of our digital age. At the same time, some valuable things have gone, or are going, by the wayside, note-taking among them. These days, students scribble on their tablets or laptops using digital styluses but rarely have subject notebooks filled with their own notes and interpretations. As a result, the need for coherent, readable notes has resurfaced and, in many of our undergraduate, graduate, and medical school classes here at the University of Vermont, we now solicit volunteer (and, sometimes, paid) notetakers specifically for this task. The intent of this short textbook is to fill that need, at least with regard to the physiology of human reproduction.

The notes are prefaced by a numbered list of close to 200 key concepts and terms. These are meant to be used as a tool: if you did not quite get a particular concept such as spermiogenesis (#34), for example, or the positive feedback mechanism underlying the LH surge (#97), you can simply skim through the list for the subject of interest, note its number, and quickly find it in the text, since the key topics are numbered sequentially and are highlighted in *blue ink* throughout. This allows you to approach the topic comprehensively by reading the entire section, or in a more targeted way by searching specific concepts. Either way,

Physiology of Human Reproduction: Notes for Students,
First Edition. George Osol.

the text is intended to serve the same purpose: helping you learn about a fascinating area of physiology whose implications are remarkably broad, spilling over into personal, political, ethical, and legal realms, and whose functioning is essential for the continuation of our species.

1

The Adult Male

[See Appendix for a review of male reproductive anatomy.]

1.1 Three Basic Requirements for Fertility in the Male

For a man to be fertile, he must fulfill three basic requirements [1]: produce semen containing sufficient numbers of healthy sperm, achieve an erection of sufficient rigidity to enter the vagina during intercourse, and be capable of ejaculating in a way that deposits semen within the vaginal canal.

Unlike the complex cyclicity of the female, male sexual function is fairly invariant. As in the female, the male reproductive system is regulated and maintained by the endocrine system, specifically the hypothalamic–pituitary–gonadal axis. The key hormones involved include: hypothalamic gonadotropin-releasing hormone (*GnRH*), two gonadotropins (*LH, FSH*) secreted from the anterior pituitary (also called the adenohypophysis), and two androgenic sex steroids (testosterone – *T*, and its metabolite dihydrotestosterone, or *DHT*).

Physiology of Human Reproduction: Notes for Students,
First Edition. George Osol.
© 2021 John Wiley & Sons Ltd. Published 2021 by John Wiley & Sons Ltd.

1.2 Endocrinology of the Male Reproductive System

The reproductive system in both sexes is driven by the pulsatile release of GnRH from the hypothalamus. GnRH [2] has a short (less than four minutes) half-life and consists of 10 amino acids that are cleaved off of a larger molecule (pre-proGnRH) whose production is coded for by chromosome 8. Once released, the GnRH decapeptide quickly travels the few millimeters to the anterior pituitary (adenohypophysis) via a specialized capillary portal system, where it binds to pituitary cells called gonadotropes (or gonadotrophs) and stimulates the release of luteinizing hormone (LH) and follicle-stimulating hormone (FSH) [3] – two gonadotropins named for their actions in the female. Like GnRH, the gonadotropins are also released in pulses and, as the term *trophic* suggests, their function is to "nourish" (Gr), i.e. to maintain the structure and function of the testes and ovaries.

Although pulsatile release [4] of GnRH, and of LH and FSH occurs in both the male and female, the *patterns* of pulsatility differ, and are used by the body to encode their physiological actions. Like a combination of AM and FM radios, their amplitude (how much hormone is released in each pulse) and frequency (time between pulses) vary over time and changes in these parameters allow the body to orchestrate the complexity of the menstrual cycle in nonpregnant women, and to maintain testosterone secretion and reproductive function in the adult male.

Although LH and FSH are structurally different, both are glycoproteins (chains of amino acids linked to sugars). Because these complex and three-dimensional molecules are charged (polar), they are unable to cross the cell membrane and rely instead on cellular recognition via receptors expressed on the plasma membrane.

Gonadotropin binding to the cell membrane is the first messenger [5]. This event activates the receptor and turns on ionic and/or enzymatic pathways inside the cell to generate the second messengers (e.g. calcium and kinases) that regulate its various functions such as secretion, metabolism, and hormone production.

Leydig cells [6] interspersed between the seminiferous tubules (also called interstitial cells for this reason) are the primary target of LH. The hormone and the cell type having a first letter in common (**LH-L**eydig) is an easy way to remember this specificity, and the main action of LH in males [7] is to stimulate the Leydig cells to produce testosterone [8]. Once released, testosterone diffuses into a neighboring seminiferous tubule, within which sperm production occurs, and initiates *paracrine* actions on the Sertoli cells [9] that form the inner lining of each seminiferous tubule to assist in the highly ordered process of spermatogenesis that results in the creation of 100–200 million new sperm daily.

Alternatively, testosterone released from the Leydig cell can be absorbed into the bloodstream via one of the many capillaries that course between the seminiferous tubules and among the Leydig cells. Once testosterone enters the vascular compartment, it travels throughout the body to exert *endocrine* actions on many tissues such as skeletal muscle or the brain.

While there are other androgenic variants and metabolites of this steroid (the most common being DHT), all androgens have 19 carbons. In contrast, progesterone has 21, and estrogen 18. The three main types of sex steroids [10] – progestogens, androgens, and estrogens – are classified by their number of carbons. In addition, there are several steroidal enzymatic pathways by which one steroid may be converted into another. For example, testosterone can be produced from progesterone via 17α-hydroxylation followed by cleavage of two carbons, and estrogen can be made from testosterone via the process of aromatization [11], which involves the appropriately named enzyme *aromatase* (Figure 1.1).

Interestingly, aromatization occurs in some of the neurons of the male brain, so that some of the central actions of testosterone – the male sex hormone – are actually carried out via its conversion into estrogen [12], the female sex hormone. Being small and highly lipid-soluble molecules, all steroids diffuse into

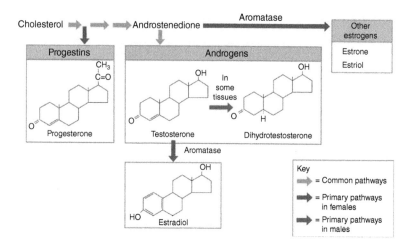

Figure 1.1 Steroidal biochemical pathways.

their target cells and enter the nucleus, where they combine with a nuclear receptor and activate or repress gene transcription. As we learn more about them, however, it is clear that there are also receptors in the cell membrane and, in the case of androgens, these are called membrane androgen receptors, or mARs. The activation of these G-protein-coupled receptors (GPCRs) leads to the generation of second messengers much like that elicited by the binding of the gonadotropins and all other peptide hormones. Acting in concert with promoter elements, testosterone modulates gene transcription to facilitate spermatogenesis and stimulates a range of Sertoli cell metabolic and secretory activities.

Once it reaches the testes, FSH [13], the other pituitary gonadotropin, diffuses from capillary across the connective tissue wall of the seminiferous tubule where it binds to the Sertoli cell membrane and elicits a cascade of second messengers. In response to FSH, Sertoli cells also make a peptide hormone of their own, called inhibin [14], which diffuses out of the tubule, enters the bloodstream and regulates FSH secretion through a negative feedback mechanism (just like testosterone regulates LH).

FSH and testosterone thereby regulate numerous Sertoli cell functions [15] in a cooperative manner. For example, Sertoli cells nurture the developing sperm by secreting nutrients (which is why they are often also called "nurture cells"). They also secrete a fluid into the lumen of the tubule that helps wash the sperm out of the tubules into the epididymis, and produce and secrete a protein called androgen-binding protein, or ABP, into the lumen of the tubule. By continually binding and releasing many testosterone molecules, ABP acts like a testosterone "sponge" and sets up a dynamic equilibrium that allows testosterone concentrations within the tubule to be as much as 50 times higher than those in the systemic circulation.

Sertoli cells also phagocytize the cellular debris shed during spermiogenesis, which we describe later, and produce immunoregulatory molecules that suppress the immune response within the seminiferous tubules. This is important, since the immune system would perceive sperm as being antigenic and mount an autoimmune response by triggering autoantibody production.

A second Sertoli-based anti-immune mechanism is physical: each individual Sertoli cell is connected to its neighbors via tight junctions, which act to "zipper" together the cells into a sheet-like intratubular barrier called the blood–testis barrier [16], preventing the passage of immune and other cells into the immunologically privileged intratubular compartment.

One final consideration related to the spatial relationships between the reproductive cells of the male and the female [17] may be helpful in remembering which hormones act on which cells. We have already considered the tripartite reproductive "unit" of the male as consisting of (i) Leydig cells outside, and (ii) Sertoli cells and (iii) sperm-forming cells inside the seminiferous tubule.

In females, the analogous reproductive units are the mature ovarian follicles. The outer follicular shell (analogous to the Leydig cells in the male) is composed of *theca cells* while the inner one (analogous to Sertoli cells) consists of *granulosa cells*. Like Leydig cells, theca cells bind LH and produce testosterone. On the other hand, the inner granulosa cells that are closest to the egg (like the Sertoli cells closest to the sperm), bind FSH and take up the testosterone released from the neighboring outer theca cells. Like Sertoli cells, granulosa cells also secrete the hormone *inhibin*, which enters the circulation and provides a negative feedback on pituitary FSH release. The one important difference is what happens to the testosterone that enters a granulosa cell: because granulosa cells have an abundance of *aromatase*, testosterone (19C) is converted to estrogen (18C) and released to diffuse out of the follicle and into the bloodstream where, and, in addition to exerting many its many endocrine effects on the uterus, brain, breasts, and other organs, the estrogen provides a negative feedback on pituitary LH release. To round out the analogy, note that Sertoli cells also contain some aromatase, and some of the Leydig cell-derived testosterone is converted into 17-beta estradiol to also help direct spermatogenesis.

1.3 Physiological Actions of Testosterone and Related Androgens

The testosterone that passes into the capillaries of the testis and circulates throughout the body has multiple and diverse endocrine actions [18] in a number of tissues. As described above, it provides a negative feedback signal to the pituitary to control LH secretion. It also regulates and maintains the structure and function of all of the associated secondary sex organs which include the various ducts (e.g. vas deferens), glands (e.g. seminal vesicles and prostate), and organs (e.g. penis, testes). Within the testis, the process of spermatogenesis would be abrogated without testosterone, and the individual would likely have a low sperm count and be infertile. A male lacking or deficient in testosterone might also experience different feelings and emotions, since testosterone is important in central nervous system (CNS) function, and would likely have a less masculine appearance and a reduced sex-drive.

Some of the most impactful actions of testosterone occur in utero [19], well before birth. If a child is destined to be a boy, testosterone production is initiated by factors derived from the Y chromosome quite early in pregnancy (weeks 6–8). Its action at this time, along with other factors secreted from the testes, is to shunt the process of sexual differentiation [20] toward the male sex by stimulating the growth of primordial male gonads and accessory ducts and glands. We initially have primitive gonads and ducts that can develop either into male or female sex organs. The Wolffian duct develops into the male; the Mullerian duct into the female. Without testosterone, the Wolffian ducts atrophy and the reproductive organs of the individual become female (default). In a male embryo, however, the female vestiges (Mullerian ducts) involute due to the secretion of anti-Mullerian hormone (secreted from the testes), while the Wolffian ducts are stimulated to grow and differentiate under the influence of testosterone, and develop into the reproductive structures of the male. This process of sexual differentiation is normally completed by week 15 of gestation.

The action of testosterone and its related androgens during and after puberty [21] is to promote growth of the secondary sexual organs like the penis and scrotum, stimulate the growth and secretory activity of the epididymis and accessory glands, and facilitate the initiation of spermatogenesis. Androgens also effect changes in the pitch of the voice (via growth of the larynx and thickening of the vocal cords), stimulate skeletal muscle development, and the development of facial, chest, and axillary hair. Testosterone stimulates protein anabolism and bone growth, although it also hastens epiphyseal closure. In the case of testosterone excess, a boy may experience accelerated growth, but end up being shorter than he would have been otherwise. In genetically prone individuals, androgens may also lead to loss of hair on the head (male pattern baldness).

After puberty, the Leydig cells of the adult male produce 6–7 mg of testosterone per day. As he passes from youth to middle, and then old age, this amount slowly declines, so that daily production is halved by the seventh or eighth decade of life.

As might be expected, this is mirrored by a similar reduction in circulating concentrations. Because this process is very gradual, however, an aging male does not undergo a sudden cessation of sex steroid production (as women do after menopause), and can remain fertile well into old age. In the adult male, testosterone stimulates the production of red blood cells (erythropoiesis), which is why men tend to have hematocrit values that are several points higher than those of women. At the same time, as circulating concentrations decrease, its physiological effects begin to wane, resulting in a slowing of metabolism, reduction in libido, and a loss of muscle mass.

Once it is absorbed into the bloodstream, testosterone circulates bound to plasma proteins, so that the effective (or "free") concentration is only 2–3% of the total hormone present in the blood. Within many tissues, testosterone functions as a prohormone, and is converted into DHT [22], an active metabolite that may be several times more potent than testosterone in its actions. The importance of DHT becomes evident when one considers the fate of individuals who lack 5α-reductase [23], the enzyme that converts T into DHT. DHT is critical for directing the normal development of the male external genitalia during embryonic life and, without it, the female structures may predominate, even though the sex is male, and underdeveloped and undescended testes may be present in the inguinal region. Hence, the individual is a genetic male (has a Y chromosome), but has the phenotypic appearance of a female.

A variation of this is the rare syndrome called androgen-insensitivity syndrome (AIS, [24]), formerly called *testicular feminization syndrome* in which a genetic male is unable to respond to testosterone due to defects on the X chromosome that result in a nonfunctional androgen receptor. When the Y chromosome stimulates the production of testosterone *in utero* during mid-pregnancy, the testosterone cannot activate its receptor and the individual will develop into a phenotypic female, e.g. he will have a vagina but no cervix or uterus, may develop breasts during puberty, and will likely be raised as a female. This individual will not be able to menstruate due to an absence of the uterus, and may only be diagnosed as an AIS patient during puberty, when the failure to menstruate becomes manifest. These days, a natural question is whether gender identity is related to sex hormone signaling and, although the field is in its infancy in terms of our understanding of its physiologic basis, there are some recent studies that have associated gender dysphoria with overrepresentation of alleles and genotypes that regulate sex-hormone signaling and responsiveness.

1.4 Spermatogenesis and Spermiogenesis

The production of healthy sperm in sufficient quantities is essential for fertility in the male. According to the World Health Organization's (WHO) latest guidelines, sperm counts [25] below 15 million/ml of semen are considered abnormal. Many men have sperm counts on the order of 50–200 million/ml of semen; therefore, it is not unusual for the total ejaculate, which has a volume of 3–5 ml, to contain more than half a billion sperm. The process of spermatogenesis is active, ongoing throughout adult life in the male, and largely genetically determined although it is also subject to influence by chemical and physical environmental factors (e.g. BPA, an estrogenic molecule found in some plastics, or heat and radiation).

Sperm produced within the seminiferous tubules [26] are transported through a series of ducts (rete testis; efferent ductules) into the epididymis. They may be stored in the epididymis or vas deferens for a considerable period of time (weeks) before passing into the urethra prior to ejaculation. The challenge of spermatogenesis is to create a sufficient number of cells that are haploid, motile, capable of penetrating the cumulus and zona pellucida of the egg, and have the ability bind to the plasma membrane of the oocyte (the oolemma).

Each testis contains hundreds of tightly packed seminiferous tubules ranging from 150 to 250 µm in diameter, and having a combined length of 30–70 cm (1–2 ft). The tubules are packed into distinct lobules, each containing one convoluted seminiferous tubule whose ends empty into a collecting region of the testes called the *rete testis.* The interior of the seminiferous tubule is lined with Sertoli cells and avascular. Sertoli cells are connected to each other by tight junctions that effectively divide each tubule into a basal (outer) and an adluminal (inner) compartment. By virtue of the blood–testis barrier, the luminal compartment is an immunologically privileged compartment free of any cells derived from the circulation. Following testicular injury or vasectomy, or in some autoimmune diseases, the production of antisperm antibodies may destroy the sperm and render the male infertile.

The progenitor cells for the production of sperm are the spermatogonia [27]. These non-differentiated cells are found in the basal compartment of the seminiferous tubules, and constantly undergo mitotic division, continually replenishing themselves. The process of spermatogenesis is initiated when some of the spermatogonia grow into primary spermatocytes [28], and migrate across the tight junctional complexes into the adluminal compartment. The mechanism involves the opening of a junction to allow a developing primary spermatocyte through, followed by its rapid closure to restore the integrity of the barrier. Once a primary spermatocyte is formed, it embarks on a spermatogenic path in which it will undergo two meiotic divisions that result in the creation of four separate haploid cells.

In the first meiotic division (*reduction division*), one primary spermatocyte forms two secondary spermatocytes [29]. Each of the two secondary spermatocytes will thus contain only 23 chromosomes, but with two copies of each due to DNA replication. The secondary spermatocyte is therefore haploid from a genetic standpoint (n rather than $2n$); however, its DNA mass is equal to that of a regular diploid cell.

Because maternal and paternal chromosomes align [30] in a random way during the first meiotic division, the chromosome present in a particular secondary spermatocyte has an equal chance of it being of either maternal or paternal origin. This presumably random event alone results in potentially more than 8 million (2^{23}) different genetic combinations just as there would be if one laid 23 coins out on a table in various heads vs. tail combinations. In addition, there is a certain degree of chromosomal mutation and translocation that occurs, particularly in prophase of the first meiotic division, resulting in an individual spawning even greater genetic diversity during spermatogenesis in the male (and, similarly, during oogenesis in the female).

Each secondary spermatocyte undergoes a second meiotic division called an *equatorial division*, in which the two secondary spermatocytes form four spermatids [31] with only one copy of each of the 23 genes per cell, i.e. haploid in terms of both genetics and DNA mass.

Once the second meiotic division is completed, the rather undistinctive appearance of each spermatid begins to undergo a morphologic change that transforms it into what we would easily recognize as a sperm. The nucleus condenses (increases in its density), and the cytoplasm is shed. The acrosome [32], a lysosome-like structure unique to spermatozoa buds from the Golgi apparatus, flattens, and comes to rest on top of the head of the sperm like a cap. The centrioles migrate to the caudal pole and form the tail by producing a long axial filament composed of nine peripheral microtubule doublets arranged around a central pair called the axoneme [33]. The axoneme is surrounded by a fibrous sheath, conferring some rigidity to the tail and is an evolutionarily conserved structure that is identical to any cilium or flagellum.

This transformation from a morphologically nonremarkable cell to the sleek and specialized motile spermatozoon (*spermatozoa* plural) is called spermiogenesis [34]. The oval head of the human sperm is only a few microns in diameter, and can exceed 50 μm in length. The acrosome capping each spermatozoon contains a variety of proteolytic enzymes such as hyaluronidase, acrosin, neuraminidase, phospholipase A, and esterases. The head of the sperm contains the tightly packed haploid DNA, and, at its caudal end, narrows to form the neck, which transitions into the midpiece. The midpiece has the axoneme in its center, and a well-organized spiral sheath of mitochondria wound around the central filament. These produce ATP to fuel locomotion via the beating of the tail, and produce energy from nutrients present in the fluid within which they are suspended. The tail propels the sperm by a twisting motion derived from interactions between tubulin fibers and dynein side arms, a process that utilizes a magnesium-dependent ATPase.

Because each spermatogonium has one X chromosome and one Y chromosome, two of the four spermatids will have a single X chromosome that will combine with the egg's X chromosome to form a genetic female, XX, and two will contain a Y chromosome which, combined with the X egg will produce a male XY genotype. The proper names for these X or Y containing sperm are gymnosperm vs. androsperm [35] based on their ability to determine the sex of the offspring. Because the Y chromosome is quite small, androsperm (Y) sperm are lighter than gymnosperm (X) and may be separated by differential centrifugation and used in assisted reproductive technology to create a baby of either sex. The sperm therefore determines the sex of the offspring.

The process of spermatogenesis is synchronized and carried out in close physical association with the Sertoli cells. The entire process is under the direct regulation of the Sertoli cell which is, in turn, guided by the combination of FSH from the pituitary, and testosterone from neighboring Leydig cells. For sperm to be functionally mature, they must pass through the epididymis, which is about an inch and a quarter in length and consists of a tightly packed, highly convoluted tube which is some 15″ in length in humans. Prior to entering the epididymis, sperm are immotile, while those exiting from the tail of the epididymis have acquired motility. A second thing of note is that sperm become decapacitated during their passage through the epididymis [36] due to the absorption of various lipids (such as cholesterol) secreted by the epididymal epithelium onto the head of the spermatozoa. This process stabilizes their membrane and is protective during ejaculation but it also renders them incapable of fertilizing the egg. Capacitation normally occurs only after ejaculation and involves a washing off of the lipids by the fluids within the female reproductive tract. Spermatozoa spend two to four weeks in the epididymis, and the entire spermatogenic process (beginning with the formation of a primary spermatocyte, two meiotic divisions, spermiogenesis, and passage through the epididymis) takes approximately 10 weeks to complete in humans.

1.5 Production of Seminal Plasma

Although the number of sperm produced daily may be staggering, spermatozoa only comprise a small fraction (about 5%) of the total ejaculate. The remaining 90–95% is composed of fluids derived from the seminal vesicles (approximately 60%), the prostate (30%), and accessory glands called the bulbourethral (or Bartholin's) glands (<5%). There are also urethral glands sprinkled along the urethra that secrete a lubricating mucus, making the walls or the penile urethra slippery and providing less resistance during ejaculation.

Prostatic secretions [37] are milky, thin, and alkaline. They contain prostate-specific antigen (PSA) which is often elevated in prostate cancer, and can therefore be used as a marker for prostatic malignancy. Prostatic secretions also contain other enzymes, most notably spermine phosphate or phosphatase, which are used as markers for semen in forensic investigation.

The secretions of the seminal vesicles [38] are sticky and rich in mucus, and contain fructose (the principal energy substrate for glycolysis in ejaculated sperm), ascorbic acid, and prostaglandins. Prostaglandins can induce smooth muscle contractility, and aid sperm ascending the female reproductive tract by inducing reverse peristalsis. They were first isolated from semen and assumed to originate in the prostate (a fact that was subsequently found not to be true), but the name has remained in use.

Finally, it is worth noting that there is also a complete clotting/declotting system [39] present in semen derived from clotting enzymes in prostatic fluid, and fibrinogen in seminal vesicle fluid. Their coordinated action during ejaculation results in the semen quickly forming a gel, affording sperm some physical protection. It also allows time for the diffusion of buffers and antibacterial substances from the coagulum into the vagina, keeps semen from leaking out of the vagina, and facilitates its ascent into the uterus and Fallopian tubes, since the reverse peristalsis is more effective against a gel than a liquid. The gel structure of semen is maintained for 15–20 minutes following ejaculation, at which time it reverts to a liquid form through a process of liquefaction [40].

1.6 Testicular Thermoregulation; Varicocoele

The human testes do not function normally at body temperature and are therefore maintained at 35 °C (~95 °F) rather than 37 °C (98.6 °F). This is accomplished by several concurrent mechanisms for testicular thermoregulation [41].

The initial event – testicular descent into the scrotum through the inguinal canal – normally occurs *in utero*, during the last trimester of pregnancy through a combination of hormonal and mechanical mechanisms. Failure of testicular descent is termed cryptorchidism (or cryptorchism; [42]), a condition that occurs in 2–3% of male infants. Failure to do so in the first few months of life warrants corrective surgery (orchiopexy) because undescended testes are associated with a 4- to 10-fold increase in the risk of developing testicular cancer, and with reduced fertility. In the adult, both testes lie within the scrotum and each is connected to the body via the spermatic cord which contains nerves, blood vessels, and the vas deferens which exit the abdominal cavity in the inguinal region. The anatomy of the inguinal region creates an area of weakness in the abdominal wall that can become herniated in response to increased intra-abdominal pressure (e.g. from straining during the Valsalva maneuver, or from lifting heavy objects). Although they can occur in women as well, 90% of the time, inguinal hernias occur in men.

Once testicular descent has occurred, the distance of the testes from the body can be regulated by a thin, sheet-like skeletal muscle called the cremaster (mechanism 1, [43]) that relaxes in a warm environment, allowing the testes to drop away from the body.

The second protective thermoregulatory mechanism involves evaporative cooling, since the scrotum is well-endowed with sweat glands (mechanism 2, [44]).

A third mechanism is countercurrent heat exchange (mechanism 3, [45]) between the testicular arteries and the veins. Blood flows down to each testis via the testicular artery, which ramifies within the testis into smaller arteries and capillaries that course between the seminiferous tubules. Blood returns from the testis via a specialized tangle of veins called the pampiniform plexus [46]. Tightly wrapped around the spermatic artery, this anatomic arrangement facilitates a countercurrent exchange of heat in which warm blood flowing to the testis is cooled by the cooler venous blood within the pampiniform plexus; conversely, the cooler venous blood returning to the body is rewarmed by the heat given up by the arterial blood within the testicular artery.

The pampiniform plexus sometimes becomes varicosed, slowing the normal flow of blood and altering testicular hemodynamics. This condition is called a varicocele [47], is not uncommon (one in six men have it to some degree) and usually (>90% of the time) occurs in the left testis. As with most varicosities, the cause is overdistension of the vein from excessive intravenous pressure.

The mechanism underlying the "sidedness" is related to an asymmetry in vascular anatomy [48]: while the right testis drains into the inferior vena cava – a large, low-pressure vessel that returns blood to the heart – the left testicular vein enters the left renal vein. Being somewhat longer than the right, and having several additional venous branches emptying into it, the left renal vein has a vigorous flow and this, in itself, creates a rheological (flow-induced) obstruction. In addition, intravenous pressure tends to be a few millimeters of mercury higher in the left vs. right renal vein because of its proximity to the superior mesenteric artery, which may compress it and impede the venous flow. This combination of high flow and increased pressure creates a backpressure that is transmitted into the pampiniform plexus, over-distending the testicular veins and resulting in permanent varicosity. Varicocele is graded based on severity and can be diagnosed by palpation, which has been likened to feeling a "bag of worms." In severe cases, it results in a softening and shrinking of the left testicle and in reducing spermatogenesis. Thus, varicocele is associated with infertility, especially if a man has a borderline sperm count. When this is a concern, varicocele can be surgically corrected by vein removal (varicocelectomy) or percutaneous embolization.

1.7 Penile Erection

Sexual arousal from physical and/or psychic stimuli results in an increase in parasympathetic drive to the reproductive organs, particularly the penis, which is largely composed of lacunar erectile tissue that is sponge-like in structure and capable of filling with blood. The efferent nerve impulses are carried to the penis by parasympathetic nerves emerging in the sacral (S2–S4) region of the spinal cord via the cavernous nerve branches of the prostatic plexus.

The penis is composed of three cords of erectile tissue [49] – the basocentral *corpus spongiosum* (which also forms the glans, or head of the penis and contains the urethra) and two *corpora cavernosa* situated in a horizontal plane above the corpus spongiosum. Note: the corpus spongiosum is sometimes referred to as the *urethral corpus cavernosum.*

The neurovascular mechanism of erection [50] during arousal involves an increased frequency of efferent parasympathetic neural impulses eliciting a release of vasodilatory neurotransmitters, particularly nitric oxide (NO) from nerves located around the small, muscular penile helicene arteries. These vessels are normally under sympathetic influence and operate in a partially constricted state (tone) that restricts the amount of blood flowing into the flaccid penis via the internal pudental artery.

During arousal, NO binds to and stimulates the enzyme *guanylate cyclase* within penile arterial smooth muscle, resulting in the conversion of *guanosine triphosphate (AGTP)* into *cyclic guanylate* monophosphate (cGMP [51]). By inducing calcium extrusion from the cell, and sequestration to intracellular organelles, cGMP reduces cytosolic calcium concentrations in arterial smooth muscle cells, decreasing force production, and leading to their relaxation and vasodilation. Blood flow increases secondary to vasodilation and the erectile tissues become engorged with blood (the filling phase, [52]), causing the penis to elongate and become tumescent.

As the erectile tissues expand secondary to the increased arterial inflow, they compress the veins, which are located peripherally, allowing maximal (nearly systemic) pressure to develop within the cavernosa and spongiosum (the tumescent phase, [53]).

Being a neurovascular process rather than a reflex (like ejaculation), erection is not all-or-none, i.e. a man may achieve partial or full erection, depending on the degree of sexual stimulation and psychological arousal. Although NO derived from nerves initiates the process, endothelial NO contributes to its maintenance. In both cases, the increase in NO results from the activation of nitric oxide synthase 3 (NO-3), which converts the amino acid arginine into citrulline, liberating NO as a byproduct.

1.8 Cellular Mechanism of PDE-5 Inhibitors in Treating Erectile Dysfunction

As with many other physiological systems, the intracellular concentration of cGMP in vascular smooth muscle reflects a summation of production (anabolism) vs. breakdown (catabolism). The breakdown of cGMP is primarily carried out by an enzyme called phosphodiesterase (PDE), and penile helicene arteries are particularly rich in the PDE-5 isoform. Inhibition of PDE-5 slows the breakdown of cGMP, favoring an increase in its cytosolic concentrations derived from NO influence. This, in turn leads to calcium extrusion from vascular smooth muscle cells and results in vasodilation.

Because drugs like sildenafil (Viagra), vardenafil (Levitra), and tadalafil (Cialis) are relatively specific PDE-5 inhibitors [54], they enhance the process of penile vasodilation and erection but do not cause it by themselves, and have much weaker effects on blood vessels in nonreproductive organs. This has some obvious practical benefits, especially for a drug like tadalafil, whose half-life is on the order of 17 hours (the half-lives of vardenafil and sildenafil are much shorter: 4–6 hours).

At the same time, some decrease in systemic blood pressure may occur because resistance arteries normally operate in a partially constricted state (tone), and their relaxation lowers peripheral resistance and blood pressure. The spillover effect is normally insignificant unless a man has very low blood pressure, or is on antihypertensive medicines, in which case PDE-5 inhibitors should be used cautiously and at the lowest dose that produces a satisfactory effect. Blood vessels of the eye have the PDE-6 isoform, which is also partially affected by PDE-5 inhibitors, and one of the less intuitive side effects of taking PDE-5 inhibitors is a change in and, very rarely, loss of vision due to nonarteritic ischemic optic neuropathy (NAION).

1.9 Emission and Ejaculation

If appropriate in pattern and of sufficient intensity, penile stimulation leads to the ejaculatory reflex [55], in which semen is expelled from the penile urethra via a sympathetic neuromuscular mechanism. Once it is triggered, ejaculation is no longer under voluntary control and is therefore most appropriately classified as a reflex.

Its efferent arc originates at the L3–L4 level where a spinal ejaculatory generator in the lumbar spinal cord stimulates a secretory center (T10–L2) that induces sequential contractions of the epididymis, vas deferens, seminal vesicles, and prostate gland.

Sperm and associated fluids from the epididymis and vas deferens are propelled into the urethra by peristaltic contractions of the vas. At the same time, the capsules of the seminal vesicles and prostate contract, increasing intraglandular pressure and forcing their secretions into the urethra. This results in the mixing of testicular/epididymal fluid containing sperm with the glandular secretions and is called the emission phase [56].

The filling of the urethra initiates sensory afferents via the pudendal nerves which travel to the mechanical center in the sacrospinal (S2–S4) region of the spinal cord and triggers the ejaculatory phase [57]. The spinal reflex mechanism induces rhythmic contractions of the striated bulbospongiosus and bulbocavernosus and ischiocavernosus muscles, propelling the semen out of the tip of the penis in spurts roughly a second apart.

Several other muscular events [58] are coordinated by the sympathetic nervous system during ejaculation. These include contraction of the neck of the bladder to prevent retrograde ejaculation, and contraction of pelvic skeletal muscles – particularly, the *ischio- and bulbo-cavernosus, and perineal muscles*, all which contribute to the pleasurable sensation of orgasm. While its occurrence is normally concurrent with ejaculation, male orgasm [59] is a physiologically distinct event which involves CNS activation, tachycardia, and acutely increased blood pressure and respiration.

1.10 Infertility

Male infertility [60] which accounts for approximately 40% of total infertility, can arise from problems with: (i) sperm number, structure, or function, (ii) obstructive disease that blocks normal emission and/or ejaculation, and (iii) disorders of sexual function. If a male does not produce sperm in sufficient concentrations, and has a low sperm count [61] (<15 million/ml of semen), he will be infertile. Similarly, if sperm are not viable, structurally abnormal, or immotile, the male may be able to achieve erection and ejaculate, but be infertile. The causes should be considered as being either pre-testicular (problems with the hypothalamo–pituitary axis or other endocrinopathies that interfere with GnRH-LH/FSH production) or testicular (e.g. a congenital absence of Sertoli cells, immune damage). Low sperm counts are the largest single cause of male infertility, and have been suggested to be responsible for up to 90% of cases.

Semen analysis [62] is a useful tool for evaluating sperm number, viability, motility, and frequency of morphologic defects. The man is asked to refrain from sexual activity for at least 48 hours, as repeated ejaculations reduce both sperm number and ejaculate volume, potentially yielding a false-positive diagnosis. Although the acrosome is not readily apparent through a light microscope, specialized stains can be applied to selectively stain for the presence of acrosomal enzymes and an intact acrosomal membrane. If problems are discovered, the cause is often endocrine in nature since spermatogenesis is ultimately dependent on the hypothalamus, pituitary, and normal Leydig and Sertoli cell function. A defect in any part of this endocrine/cellular system may be responsible for low sperm count and male factor infertility. Finally, epididymal defects that result in immotile sperm and structural defects (two heads, bent tails; absence of an acrosome; defective genetic material) may all contribute to reducing the viability of sperm and, hence, male fertility.

Parameters for semen analysis [63] are currently based on 2010 WHO guidelines, and include the 15 million/ml reference value for sperm count (39 million per total ejaculate, and a volume of at least 1.5 ml), along with >40% total motility (32% for forward progressive motility), and 58% viability. Their values are remarkably forgiving for one parameter in particular: morphology; for a semen sample to be considered normal, only 4% of sperm have to appear normal.

The second broad cause of male infertility is obstruction. This may be due to a congenital absence of vas deferens, for example, from scarring following trauma or infection, or from a voluntary surgical procedure such as vasectomy. A variant, hypospadias [64], is due to an anatomical anomaly in which the urethra exits the penis at its base rather than tip. In this case, there is no obstruction, *per se* – rather, the inability to deposit sperm in the vaginal canal, precluding normal insemination.

The third category of male infertility is *sexual dysfunction*, e.g. an inability to produce an erection or to ejaculate. The underlying causes are numerous, and may be psychological, neural, vascular, or muscular in origin. The older term – *impotence* – has been replaced in recent years by erectile dysfunction (ED, [65]), defined as *the inability of a male to produce an erection of sufficient rigidity to deposit semen intravaginally*. As already discussed, these days, ED is most often aided by oral PDE-5 inhibitors such as sildenafil. Neural or vascular damage may also lead to sexual dysfunction, in which case PDE-5 inhibition may be of limited use. ED be due to many different causes, including spinal cord injury, autonomic and peripheral neuropathy, endocrine disorders, psychogenic disorders (e.g. performance anxiety and depression), atherosclerosis (yes, it can occur there too), and drug-induced effects. Anything that affects the neurovascular pathway we already discussed may affect sexual function, even physical compression (as in poorly designed bicycle seats). Ironically, while depression can lower libido, so can antidepressant drugs (such as Prozac).

One last word on impotence vs. infertility [66]. The former term is narrower than the latter, and is defined as "the consistent inability to achieve or sustain an erection of sufficient rigidity for sexual intercourse". A summary of causes of male infertility can be found in Table 1.1, below.

Table 1.1 Causes of Male Infertility

I. Disorders of spermatogenesis

A. Pre-testicular (e.g. pituitary and endocrine disorders, tumors)
B. Testicular (e.g. varicocele, cryptorchidism)

II. Obstruction of the efferent ducts

A. Congenital (e.g. absence of the vas deferens)
B. Acquired (e.g. vasectomy)

III. Disorders of sperm motility

A. Congenital (immotile Cilia syndrome, epididymal dysfunction)
B. Acquired (antisperm antibodies)

IV. Sexual dysfunction

A. Congenital (immotile Cilia syndrome, epididymal dysfunction)
B. Impotence
C. Ejaculatory abnormalities (e.g. retrograde ejaculation)

2

The Nonpregnant Adult Female

[See Appendix for a review of female reproductive anatomy.]

2.1 The Menstrual Cycle: A Perspective

Puberty in girls leads to the initiation of monthly menstrual cycles (beginning with the first cycle called the menarche [67]). Every textbook has a menstrual cycle that is exactly 28 days long (equal to the lunar month), and so do many women. At the same time, menstrual cycle length [68] within a population of women can vary considerably, with cycles as short as 20 days and as long as 40 days having been reported. An intriguing, but poorly understood phenomenon is the "sorority house syndrome" in which the menstrual cycles of young women who live together somehow come to be synchronous. The mechanism is not understood, but likely involves pheromones or other environmental and social cues.

While anecdotal, this example serves to illustrate a simple truth – that the physiological mechanisms that govern the menstrual cycle are responsive to and can be influenced by a number of internal and external factors, including diet, exercise, environment, and stress. If a woman's body fat content decreases beyond a certain point, for example, her menstrual cycles may become irregular or cease.

Physiology of Human Reproduction: Notes for Students,
First Edition. George Osol.
© 2021 John Wiley & Sons Ltd. Published 2021 by John Wiley & Sons Ltd.

The menstrual cycle is driven by the hypothalamic pulse generator [69], which begins to send out pulses of GnRH that stimulate the secretion of FSH and luteinizing hormone (LH; also pulsatile) from the anterior pituitary. Over the course of the menstrual cycle, the character (frequency and amplitude) of the pulses changes, an observation that suggests an encoding phenomenon based on their pattern of release. At this point, you might ask, encoding of what? To answer that question, let us consider what has to happen, and where.

The menstrual cycle is a highly coordinated physiological process that involves the brain (hypothalamus, pituitary) stimulating the development of a small group of follicles in each ovary every month, one of which will become a mature follicle and rupture mid-month through the process of ovulation, releasing an oocyte usually destined to end up in the neighboring fallopian tube. If the conditions are right, this oocyte may be fertilized to begin a pregnancy although the postovulatory window for fertilization is short – on the order of 16–20 hours.

Let us begin by considering oogenesis – the production of oocytes via a process whose purpose is similar to that of spermatogenesis: the production of a haploid cell. The timing, pattern, and nature of the process, however, are quite different.

2.2 Oogenesis

If a child is destined to be female, the absence of a Y chromosome prevents the production of testosterone during embryonic life. Without it, the system follows the default path, i.e. the development of a female reproductive system. This entails growth of the Mullerian (primordial female) ducts and involution of the Wolffian (primordial male) ducts [70], and leads to the development of the female gonads – the ovaries.

Beginning around week six of pregnancy, primordial germ cells destined to become oocytes form within the embryonic yolk sac, migrate to the genital ridge, and become incorporated into the surface of the developing ovaries to form a germinal epithelium [71]. Their formation and migration into the ovarian cortex are followed by differentiation to form oogonia [72], which continue to proliferate by mitosis between weeks 5 and 10 of gestation. Some of these oogonia begin to transform into primary oocytes [73] by commencing meiosis so that, by midpregnancy, all of the oogonia have transformed into primary oocytes which are no longer capable of undergoing mitosis and can therefore no longer be replenished.

During the second half of pregnancy, the number of primary oocytes begins to decrease through a process of attrition [74]. Thus, there may be 1–2 million primary oocytes at the time of birth, a few hundred thousand by the time a girl reaches puberty, and 10–30 000 by the time the woman is in her mid-30s. Eventually, by the time a woman enters her sixth decade, the number of oocytes is reduced to zero, at which point her monthly cycles cease, and she becomes menopausal.

Like a primary spermatocyte, the primary oocyte must undergo two meiotic divisions to become haploid. The first meiotic division begins *in utero*, when the oogonium grows into the primary oocyte, arresting in prophase of the first meiotic division. Here, it may be helpful to remember the phases of meiosis by a somewhat clumsy but useful acronym: *IPMAT* (*I*nterphase, *P*rophase, *M*etaphase, *A*naphase, and *T*elophase). Once an oogonium becomes a primary oocyte, it can no longer undergo mitosis, and the meiotic process is then paused until puberty. Afterward, the primary oocyte may complete its first meiotic division and become a secondary oocyte [75], but only if it is recruited during a particular cycle. Like the secondary spermatocyte, the secondary oocyte is genetically haploid, having 23 chromosomes, but with two copies of each. The secondary spermatocyte begins its second meiotic division but then arrests in metaphase [76]. The second meiotic division *will only be completed if that secondary oocyte is ovulated and fertilized by a sperm*, at which point it becomes the ovum [77].

Unlike the male, where one primary spermatocyte forms two secondary spermatocytes, when the primary oocyte undergoes the first meiotic division, one of the daughter cells becomes a secondary oocyte while the other is a small, nonfunctional structure called a polar body [78]. If it is fertilized, the secondary oocyte completes the second meiotic division to become an ovum, and a second polar body is extruded in the process. Another way of looking at it is that all of the energy is put into creating one egg cell rather than four, since only one oocyte is normally ovulated during a particular menstrual cycle. Accordingly, it is a very large cell that is more than 100 microns in diameter (whereas most cells are only 5-10 microns in diameter).

2.3 Folliculogenesis

Once it has formed *in utero*, every primary oocyte comes to be surrounded by a single layer of flattened cells called granulosa cell precursors [79]. This simple, small (~30 μm diameter) structure is called the unilaminar or primordial follicle [80]. The total number of primordial follicles begins to decline through a process of follicular attrition as already described in the previous section on oogenesis, such that 70–80% of the primordial follicles may involute before a girl is born.

The number of primordial follicles continues to decrease through childhood, puberty, and during the reproductive life of a woman, which is on the order of 40 years. Most women's ovaries become completely depleted of follicles in the sixth decade of life, and her menstrual cycles cease. At this point, she is no longer capable of becoming pregnant and, once she has not had a menstrual cycle for a year, she will be considered to be menopausal. The transition from having normal cycles to not cycling at all takes several years as menstrual cycles become less regular and frequent; this transitional period is referred to as the female climacteric.

As in the male, postpubescent pulsatile GnRH release stimulates the release of the two gonadotropins in the female – LH and FSH – from anterior pituitary gonadotrophs and these, in turn, activate the female reproductive system by inducing ovarian changes that lead to the monthly cycle of events that we call the menstrual cycle.

The ovary responds to FSH in an usual way. Rather than being uniformly stimulated, as one might expect, only a small group of primordial follicles begin to grow and develop into primary follicles [81] every month. This group, numbering perhaps a dozen or more, is termed a *cohort*, and is selected through the still poorly understood process of follicular recruitment [82] that actually begins many months before and involves cytological changes in the oocyte, follicular cells, and adjacent connective tissues.

The flat, squamous shell of pre-granulosa cells becomes cuboidal, or even columnar, and undergoes mitosis to form a multilayered stratified epithelium. The oocyte enlarges, and its cytoplasm changes in character – there are more free ribosomes, the endoplasmic reticulum proliferates, and vesicles form just under the plasma membrane (oolemma). The oocyte membrane becomes microvillous and secretes an amorphous material that becomes the zona pelucida [83] – an acellular, gel-like glycoprotein layer that coats the oocyte. Meanwhile, a sheath of stromal cells grows around the granulosa cell sphere to form the thecal layer, which develops an inner (*theca interna*) and an outer (*theca externa*) portion. The granulosa–theca border is demarcated by a basement membrane, and small blood vessels grow into the theca, forming a rich capillary plexus. The granulosa layer, however, remains completely avascular, as vessels are unable to pass beyond the basement membrane.

During a period of approximately two weeks, the primary follicle develops into a secondary follicle [84]. The latter is also called an antral follicle because it is characterized by the appearance of a fluid-filled cavity around the oocyte (the *antrum*). As the follicle continues to grow, the oocyte – surrounded by the zona pellucida – comes to be perched on a pedestal of granulosa cells that secrete, and are bathed in a rich fluid called the follicular fluid, or *liquor folliculi* [85]. As the term liquor implies, it is strong stuff (at least in terms of hormonal concentrations, which can be >100× higher than those in the circulation). Estrogen, the primary female sex steroid hormone, is produced and secreted by the granulosa cells.

The cohort of secondary follicles continue to grow, and one eventually outpaces the others to become the tertiary (also called the dominant, vesicular, mature, or Graafian follicle [86]). At this point, the tertiary follicle is the primary source of estrogen and is visible to the eye during laparoscopic surgery, as it attains a diameter of 4–5 mm (1/4") prior to ovulation. As such, it is approximately 100–150× larger than the primordial follicle from which it developed. If we scale the primary follicle up to the size of a basketball, the mature follicle would be represented by a sphere some 10 or 15 stories high! Since the individual cells are of a similar size, you can imagine the extent of cell division required to produce such a large, beautifully organized spherical structure during an approximately two-week period.

This initial phase of the menstrual cycle during which a cohort of follicles is induced to grow, and which terminates with the formation of a mature tertiary follicle (that will shortly rupture during the process of ovulation) is called – from the standpoint of the ovary, since that is where all this is happening – the follicular phase [87]. At the same time, there are events going on in the uterus (which we consider below) and, as you will see, it is important to distinguish the ovarian phases from the uterine phases of the menstrual cycle as they are completely different. At the same time, they are interconnected since the ovary controls the uterus through its secretion of steroid hormones: estrogen during the first half of the cycle, and estrogen and progesterone during the second half.

The length of the *follicular phase* [88] may be quite variable from woman to woman, and it accounts for most of the variability in the length of a menstrual cycle. When one considers how we each have our own individual growth patterns, this is not surprising. Conversely, the second half of the ovarian cycle, during which the shell of the ovulated follicle is transformed into the corpus luteum (CL) is much less variable and almost always 14 days in length. This is because the death of the CL is programmed to occur two weeks after its formation shortly after ovulation. Hence, a woman with a menstrual cycle that is 20 days long probably has a follicular phase that is likely only 6 days long; conversely, someone with a 34-day cycle has a follicular phase that is likely 20 (34 minus 14) days long.

2.4 Follicular Production of Sex Steroid Hormones

As already mentioned above, the main hormone produced and secreted by the growing follicle is estrogen [89]. This critical endocrine event is largely under the influence of LH, the other pituitary gonadotropin. Most simply, FSH stimulates follicles to grow while LH stimulates their production and secretion of estrogen via a cooperative mechanism [90] between the theca and granulosa cells.

Substrates like cholesterol delivered via the bloodstream are taken up by the theca cells that comprise the outer shell of an antral follicle. These cells possess a large number of LH receptors and contain steroidogenic enzymes that catalyze the production of testosterone [91]. Once it is synthesized, the testosterone is released from the theca cell, and diffuses across the basement membrane into the inner part of the follicle (granulosa cell layer and oocyte) where it exerts a paracrine action.

As already noted, this is spatially akin to the Leydig–Sertoli cell arrangement in the male (relative to the location of the germ cells) since Leydig cells are on the outside, while Sertoli cells are inside the seminiferous tubule (which also has a basement membrane within its wall).

The granulosa cells aromatize the androgen into estrogen [92], which is then released into the follicular fluid inside the follicle, where it can accumulate. Some estrogen also diffuses back into the thecal cell layer, which is vascularized, allowing it to pass into the systemic circulation. The amount of estrogen produced by any particular follicle is dependent on the number of cells producing it, i.e. its size. It is therefore not surprising then that the biggest follicle (eventually, the mature or tertiary follicle) will produce the most estrogen. The question is: how does it become the biggest, i.e. how is it recruited?

2.5 Recruitment of the Dominant Follicle

As already discussed, a small cohort [93] of primordial follicles in each ovary begins to grow and develop into primary, and then secondary (antral) follicles during each menstrual cycle. How this particular cohort is chosen is anybody's guess. Suffice it to say that the process begins months earlier through an ill-defined process of selection and recruitment spurred on by FSH.

As this month's recruited follicular cohort begins to grow (normally, a handful of follicles in each ovary), the granulosa cells within each begin to secrete estrogen, which is absorbed into the bloodstream and exerts a negative feedback effect on the brain that diminishes LH secretion from the pituitary. The granulosa cells of each developing follicle also secrete inhibin, which decreases the secretion of FSH. This is a bit of an oversimplification, since there are at least five different hormones involved in this process involving the inhibin–activin family [94] – peptide hormones; as the name implies, each exerts its own particular effects at the local and systemic level. For example, inhibin B has negative feedback effects only on FSH secretion, while inhibin A is believed to inhibit both LH and FSH. This family of hormones is present in both males and females, and is still not well understood. Activin actions are also multiple, one of which is to regulate FSH and LH actions on the follicle.

A fraction of the estrogen produced by each follicle passes into the systemic circulation and exerts endocrine effects on the brain and other (e.g. reproductive) organs. It also has some local (paracrine/autocrine) effects within the follicle, e.g. increasing its responsiveness to FSH via the induction of new FSH receptors.

During the follicular phase, one of the follicles pulls ahead of the others to become the dominant follicle [95] which is larger (and therefore more secretory) than the rest because it has more estrogen-producing cells. As it produces more and more estrogen and inhibin, pituitary LH and FSH secretion is further suppressed, slowing the growth of the other follicles within that particular cohort. Occasionally, two follicles may emerge as being dominant, and two oocytes may be ovulated. If both are ovulated and fertilized, fraternal twins will develop.

2.6 Transition from the Follicular to the Ovulatory Phase: The LH Surge

Once the dominant follicle has formed, its next task is to undergo the process of rupture, or ovulation. This is no small feat, and requires a mechanism that is specific, unique, and endocrine in nature. The challenge is met through a clever variation of normal endocrine physiology.

As follicles grow, estrogen concentrations in the bloodstream increase progressively through the follicular phase [96]. As already noted, once a dominant follicle is present, it suppresses the production of estrogen by other follicles (and of LH via negative feedback), but continues to produce its own estrogen in increasing amounts, so that circulating concentrations continue to increase. One can view this phase as being one where the dominant follicle is on autopilot, as it somehow escapes the consequences of decreasing LH (and FSH) levels and keeps rapidly growing and secreting estrogen from the granulosa cell layer.

When circulating estrogen concentrations increase beyond approximately 300 pg/ml, an unusual thing occurs. Rather than inhibiting LH release, the feedback mechanism "flips" from being negative to positive, i.e. rather than inhibiting pituitary LH, estrogen begins to stimulate LH secretion (Figure 2.1).

The unusual nature of this event deserves a special name, and the one that has been used for decades to convey its magnitude is: the LH surge [97]. Like a storm surge at sea, LH

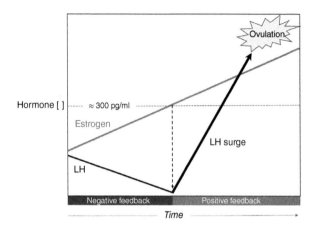

Figure 2.1 Increasing estrogen concentrations trigger LH surge via positive feedback on the anterior pituitary, leading to ovulation.

levels rise and crest and, as they do, the secretion of the liquor folliculi by the granulosa cells increases. As more follicular fluid is secreted into the antrum, the intrafollicular pressure begins to rise. At the same time, the matrix between the follicular cells weakens, eventually leading to the rupture of the follicle (ovulation) and the release of the secondary oocyte and its surrounding granulosa cells from the surface of the ovary. This represents the *ovulatory phase* [98].

Because ovulation is predicated on the progressive increase in LH levels, and because this LH surge occurs over a period of 24–36 hours prior to ovulation, measuring LH levels would be a good way to predict ovulation. Circulating levels are difficult to assess, however, because they are pulsatile and change minute-to-minute. Also, a commercial ovulation detection test using circulating LH concentrations would require repeated blood drawings, a process that is invasive and unpleasant.

Luckily, LH is filtered by the kidneys and secreted into the urine, providing an easily accessible fluid for analysis and one that reflects an averaged, rather than momentary concentration index. Ovulation detection kits [99], which are available over-the-counter in most pharmacies, take advantage of this approach and, by virtue of their detection of urinary LH, allow a couple to plan their sexual activity to coincide with the period of highest female fertility. Once the egg is released from the follicle, it is only fertilizable for less than a day, hence, knowing that you will be ovulating within the next 12, 24, or 36 hours provides very useful (and actionable!) physiological "intelligence" for a couple seeking to have a child.

2.7 The Luteal Phase

The process of ovulation ruptures the pedestal that the oocyte sits on within the follicle thereby releasing the secondary oocyte along with a clump of surrounding granulosa cells. These oocyte-surrounding granulosa cells are important in guiding the nutrition and maturation of the oocyte within the follicle and are collectively called the cumulus oophorus [100]. Once the egg has been ovulated, a number of cumulus (granulosa) cells remain attached to the oocyte, surrounding it and the zona pellucida layer just beyond the oolemma (plasma membrane of the oocyte). This entire structure (oocyte, zona, granulosa cells) looks like a crown and is called the corona radiata [101].

At the time of ovulation, the distal end of the oviduct, which widens into finger-like projections called the fimbriae, comes to lie close to the ovary and, once the oocyte–granulosa complex is ejected from the follicle, it is swept into the oviduct by the ciliary motion of the widened (fimbriated) end of the oviductal epithelium and begins to pass down the oviduct toward the uterus.

But what about the shell of the follicle that remains in the ovary? The theca and many granulosa cells are still there, and they undergo a morphological and biochemical transformation under the influence of LH. The remnant of the follicle becomes reorganized into a fatty-appearing, but very active gland that contains a mixture of large and small cells (derived from the granulosa and theca cells) that lacks the distinct, spatially defined morphology of the Graafian follicle. This new structure on the surface of the ovary is called the corpus luteum, or CL [102] (yellow body). Its yellowness reveals the fact that it is an active steroidogenic endocrine gland that continues to make estrogen, but also secretes increasing amounts of another female sex steroid – progesterone [103]. As the name implies, progesterone is the progestational hormone that is essential for pregnancy. The hormone that stimulates the transformation of the ruptured follicle into the CL is, not surprisingly, LH (luteinizing hormone). This transformation of the remaining follicular shell on the surface of the ovary into the CL occurs immediately after ovulation and begins the second half of the ovarian cycle termed the *luteal phase* [104].

Keep in mind that, thus far, we have only been focused on the events that occur in the ovary. These can be summed up in three OVARIAN phases: (i) the *follicular phase*, in which follicles grow under the influence of FSH and a dominant follicle emerges, (ii) the *ovulatory phase*, which occurs at the approximate midpoint of the menstrual cycle (day 14 in textbooks), and in which the egg and its vestments (corona radiata) are extruded from the ovary into the fallopian tube, and (iii) the *luteal phase*, in which the follicular shell transforms into the CL, an endocrine gland that produces increasing amounts of progesterone, along with some estrogen. A natural question at this point might be – why bother to make all that estrogen and progesterone?

2.8 Corresponding Uterine Phases: Menstrual, Proliferative, Secretory

The answer to this question requires us to think about what must happen for pregnancy to begin and progress normally, and this line of inquiry leads directly to the uterus.

The uterus is a compact muscular organ that is largely made up of smooth muscle (the myometrium). But it is its thin and highly specialized inner lining – the endometrium [105] – that is essential for fertility, and key to understanding early pregnancy physiology. Although the musculature is critical for carrying out labor, it is the endometrium that provides the proper environment for implantation and subsequent embryonic and fetal development.

The concept of a field provides a good working analogy. If you want to grow corn, you need earth to grow it in. More accurately, you need topsoil, a rich mixture of organic matter that can provide the nutrients required to sprout a seed and support its growth into a mature plant.

The endometrium can be viewed as the "field of pregnancy." Without it, pregnancy cannot succeed, and therefore its proper cellular and vascular organization and function are essential for supporting gestation. As you might suspect, this aspect is not controlled haphazardly. The ovary – under the influence of the brain – guides and manages the uterus to a high degree by jettisoning the endometrium of the last cycle (menstruation), stimulating its *de novo* growth, and fine-tuning its transformation into a structure that secretes nutrients to help nurture the blastocyst (uterine milk), and to facilitate its implantation. During the course of pregnancy, ovarian steroids also affect the myometrium by stimulating changes in its vascular smooth muscle cells and connective tissue to favor growth and accommodation of the fetoplacental unit, and by enhancing contractile function in preparation for labor.

The only mechanism available to the ovary, which is physically separate and distinct from the uterus, and not connected to it by nerves, is to utilize an endocrine mechanism, since the only physiological connection available to it is via the circulation. Therefore, the ovary controls the endometrium via the two sex steroid hormones that we have already discussed – estrogen and progesterone. Let us work through a new menstrual cycle, this time focusing on what happens in the uterus rather than the ovary. The first challenge is to get rid of the last month's endometrium via the process of menstruation.

The menstrual phase [106] is triggered by the death of the CL, which leads to a sharp drop in circulating levels of estrogen and progesterone. Since it is self-evident (unlike ovulation, for example, or the time when a new cohort of follicles begins to grow), the first day of menstruation is used to mark the beginning of a new menstrual cycle. Parenthetically, it is also used to date pregnancy since a woman may not know when she ovulates, but she is normally aware of when she last menstruated. The process of menstruation reduces the thickness of the endometrium, from 14 to 15 mm to perhaps 2 or 3 mm.

Normally, the menstrual phase lasts about five days, therefore, it comprises days 1–5 of the menstrual cycle from the standpoint of the uterus, and coincides with the first part of the follicular phase in the ovary. Like the length of a menstrual cycle, the number of days a woman menstruates also varies from three to eight days, and can be affected by external influences, particularly, oral or depo methods of birth control. Once the old endometrium is shed, the new one begins to grow under the influence of estrogen coming from this month's cohort of follicles, and the end of menstruation therefore marks the beginning of the second uterine phase: *the proliferative phase* [107].

During this period, under the influence of estrogen coming from the cohort of developing follicles, the endometrium grows through a process of cellular proliferation, increasing in thickness from 1–2 to 9–10 mm by the time of ovulation (day 14 in a 28-day cycle). Following ovulation, once the CL is formed, progesterone stimulates a transformation of the endometrium into a secretory structure by inducing the development and secretory activity of numerous uterine glands that form during the first half of the cycle, but mature and become active in the second half. For this reason, the second half of the menstrual cycle (from the standpoint of the uterus) is called *the secretory phase* [108].

If pregnancy has not occurred, it is important to get rid of the old endometrium and start growing a new one during the next menstrual cycle. This is effected by the death of the CL [109], which is timed to occur two weeks after its postovulatory formation. The exact mechanism in humans in not well-understood, but in a number of other mammalian species, prostaglandins released by the uterus are transferred from uterine veins to the ovarian arteries (which are adjacent), and the prostaglandins act to constrict the blood vessels leading to the CL, inducing ischemia and necrosis. On the other hand, if fertillization occurs and a pregnancy takes, the death of the CL is unacceptable, since the ensuing menstruation would lead to an ejection of the implanted embryo with the menstrual flow. The CL must therefore be rescued by the embryo [110], and the mechanism involves secretion of human chorionic gonadotropin (hCG), an LH-like hormone, by the embryo. The hCG keeps the CL functioning until the embryo and its placenta make sufficient estrogen and progesterone to no longer have to rely on the CL (an event termed the luteo-placental shift and which occurs around weeks 7–8 of human pregnancy).

2.9 Estrogen

Estrogen is a powerful hormone that affects nearly every organ in the body. It currently enjoys a mixed reputation, since it is associated with youth and fertility on the one hand, and some forms of cancer and, more recently, an increased likelihood of unfavorable cardiovascular events (stroke, thrombosis) when administered orally after menopause on the other.

As a steroid, estrogen is lipid-soluble and can easily diffuse into cells. Although it does have some non-genomic effects on the membrane, most of its actions occur secondary to its binding to nuclear receptors. Two estrogen receptors [111] – ERα and ERβ – have been identified. They share some structural homology, but are for the most part quite different both in terms of their molecular structure, tissue distribution, and function.

Some of the major actions of estrogen [112] in the nonpregnant female include:

- Expression of female secondary sex characteristics during puberty and, thereafter, maintenance of female reproductive structures, in particular, the ovaries, oviducts, uterus,

and breasts (particularly lactiferous ducts), and maintenance of vaginal structure and secretory functions.

- Exerting endocrine feedback actions on the hypothalamus and pituitary, especially in regulating the secretion
of LH (both negative and positive mechanisms exist, as
you now know).
- Stimulating the growth and vascularization of the endometrium during the menstrual cycle, and preparing the
endometrium for the actions of progesterone by inducing
the production of progesterone receptors within the endometrial stroma.
- Stimulating watery secretions from the cervix that facilitate ascending sperm transport into the uterus (this has
a spillover anti-acne effect because of a similar effect on
sebaceous glands, reducing the chances of developing
pimples from clogged sebaceous gland ducts).
- Contributing to the maintenance and progression of pregnancy, particularly in terms of maternal cardiovascular
and hematologic adaptation.
- Exerting protective cardiovascular effects.

In addition, estrogen affects cognitive and CNS functions,
maintains bone function and density, and mediates a range of
other feminizing actions. The importance of its actions become
evident when a woman goes through menopause and thereafter
faces many health risks secondary to the loss of estrogen, e.g.
increased incidence of cardiovascular disease and osteoporosis.

2.10 Progesterone

Being a steroid, progesterone, like estrogen, binds to receptors
found in the nuclei of many different kinds of cells. A commonly overlooked fact is that it is actually secreted throughout
the menstrual cycle, but in much greater amounts during the
second half (luteal phase).

The major actions of progesterone [113] include:

- Stimulating endometrial and cervical secretions. Unlike estrogen, progesterone induces the production of thick, mucous secretions that seal off the lower end of the uterus for pregnancy (this is called the cervical plug in some animals, but is not nearly as dense in humans). The effect on sebaceous glands promotes the development of acne during the luteal phase.
- Stimulating the growth of the myometrium during pregnancy.
- Exerting a pacifying influence on smooth muscle, leading to the quiescence of the uterus during pregnancy, and a reduction in the motility of the oviducts.
- Stimulation of the growth of the breasts during puberty and during pregnancy (particularly of the glandular tissue).
- If progesterone levels are too low, a woman's fertility may decrease since the endometrium is not adequately prepared for implantation. This condition, called luteal phase defect, may contribute to infertility and can be treated by oral progesterone in the second half of the cycle.

2.11 Putting It Together

As you can see, the menstrual cycle can only be understood from the standpoint of the organs that are key to its coordination, and these are principally the ovaries and uterus. The hypothalamus and pituitary are important as well, but ultimately it is the ovary that seems to have the most central control.

We talked about the three ovarian phases – the follicular phase (days 1–14), the ovulatory phase (day 14), and the luteal phase (days 14–28).

Within the uterus, there are also three phases. Phase 1 is the menstrual phase (days 1–5), during which the endometrium of the last cycle is extruded. At this point, the ovary is already in the follicular phase, and the cohort of follicles destined to develop during this month has begun to develop. Uterine Phase 2 is the proliferative phase (days 5–14), during which endometrial

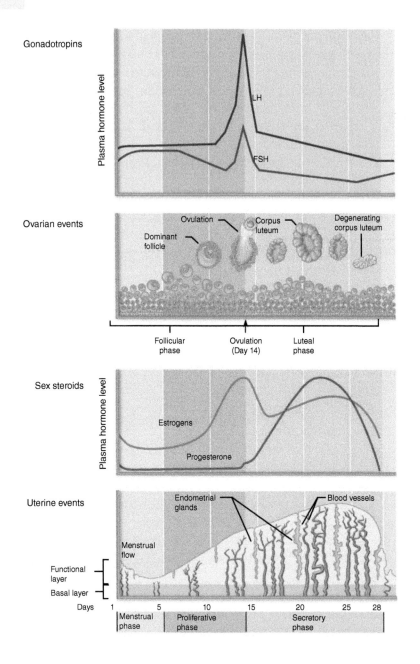

Figure 2.2 Key events associated with the menstrual cycle.

thickness, vascularity and organization increases progressively under the influence of ovarian estrogen. Uterine Phase 3 corresponds to the luteal phase in the ovary, and is called the secretory phase (days 15–28), during which progesterone coming from the CL stimulates the secretory activity of the uterine glands, and estrogen maintains endometrial integrity. During the second half of the cycle, the endometrial glands secrete a fluid called "uterine milk" into the uterine lumen. This fluid is thought to nourish the blastocyst, assist its implantation, and suppress the maternal immune system, thereby avoiding allogeneic rejection of the embryo (due to the presence of paternally inherited antigens). The figure above provides a coordinated summary of the key hormonal changes and ovarian and uterine events across one menstrual cycle (Figure 2.2).

3 Pregnancy, Parturition, Lactation

3.1 Fertilization and Early Embryogenesis

During intercourse, a man normally ejaculates hundreds of millions of sperm into the vaginal canal. For fertilization to occur, the male and female germ cells (gametes) must come into close proximity and, eventually, direct contact. Several specialized physiological mechanisms facilitate their encounter within the relative vastness of the tubal lumen.

Around the time of ovulation, the fimbriated (widened) distal end of the oviduct is drawn closer to the ovary. This movement has been described as "enveloping" or even "caressing" the ovary. The infundibular (and fallopian) epithelium is ciliated and, by beating in a directional wave-like pattern, the secondary oocyte and its vestments [114] are swept into and down the fallopian tube. Unlike the rapid ascent by sperm, this is a much slower process, as an egg, if fertilized, takes close to a week to pass through the fallopian tube and enter the uterine lumen.

The ovulated oocyte itself would be difficult to discern at this time, as it is coated with an acellular soft glycoprotein layer (the zona pellucida) which is, in turn, surrounded by an adherent cumulus of granulosa cells (corona radiata, [115]).

Physiology of Human Reproduction: Notes for Students,
First Edition. George Osol.
© 2021 John Wiley & Sons Ltd. Published 2021 by John Wiley & Sons Ltd.

The secondary oocyte is a very large cell ($\approx$100 μm in diameter, some 10× larger than a typical somatic cell) and, because it is surrounded by the zona pellucida and corona radiata of granulosa cells, its overall diameter is on the order of 200–300 μm. Granulosa cells provide nourishment and supply vital proteins to the secondary oocyte; once it has been ovulated, the surrounding cells may also play some functional role, although this aspect is not well understood.

The secondary oocyte must encounter a sperm within a day of fertilization, since it is only capable of being fertilized for 16–20 hours, after which time it disintegrates and is reabsorbed. Human sperm, on the other hand, can survive in the female reproductive tract for several days, and so the window of pregnancy [116] in the human female is approximately four to five days long, beginning three to four days prior to ovulation (the exact time is dependent on the physiological properties of the male sperm and its disposition with the female reproductive tract) and postovulatory day 1.

Let us say a man and a woman have sexual intercourse and his ejaculate contains 500 million sperm suspended in a volume of several milliliters of semen. During and immediately after ejaculation, millions of sperm die because of mechanical damage, the acidity of the female reproductive tract, or due to the presence of other factors such as bacteria, proteolytic enzymes, etc. Because of this, the number of viable sperm [117] that pass through the cervix into the uterus is actually a tiny fraction of that which was initially ejaculated and, by some estimates, only 1–2% are still alive a few minutes after ejaculation.

As discussed in Section 1.5, the ejaculate quickly coagulates into a gel that liquefies some 20–25 minutes later. This process of semen coagulation followed by liquefaction [118] serves to protect the sperm, since the fluid part of semen (the sperm cells only comprise ~5% of the seminal volume) contains a number of substances that are helpful to sperm survival. These include antibiotics, buffers that neutralize vaginal acidity, and nutrients that diffuse out of the gel while the sperm are still trapped within. The physical properties of the gel and some of its components (e.g. prostaglandins) stimulate reverse peristalsis within the female reproductive tract, thereby facilitating the transport of sperm up through the cervical canal and into the uterus and fallopian tubes.

At the midpoint of the menstrual cycle, when ovulation occurs, the cervix widens, and its secretions become quite thin and watery due to the predominance of estrogen. Mucin molecules in the cervical mucus [119] become oriented parallel to each other, forming channels that favor sperm migration. In addition, cervical crypts formed by the infolding of columnar endocervical epithelium provide spaces for sperm to accumulate, and from which they may be slowly released over time to ascend into the uterus. In some avian species (turkeys, for example), this is quite dramatic, as sperm can be released for weeks on end, and the cervical crypts have accordingly been called "sperm nests."

At the same time, sperm have been detected in the fallopian tube, and even in the abdominal cavity minutes after intercourse. Although they are capable of swimming some 25 μm/sec, unassisted, the distance sperm must travel (4–5", or approximately 12 cm) would take them an hour or more to traverse. Clearly, they are getting some help in moving along and, in this case, the assist mechanism is reverse peristalsis [120] induced by the prostaglandins present in semen. As a result, the loose seminal coagulum is pushed up into the upper third of the uterus and into the lumen of the oviducts.

Of the fifty to a few hundred million sperm present in the typical ejaculate, only a few thousand likely reach the vicinity of the egg due to the relative vastness of the tubal lumen, the fact that some sperm may end up in the oviduct that does not contain an egg, and because uterine reverse peristalsis is only modestly efficient.

Here, one might wonder whether there is some kind of a selection process that determines which sperm finally fertilizes the egg? The likelihood of a physiological process for sperm selection, at least in terms of genetic quality, is undermined by the fact that 60–75% of human pregnancies terminate spontaneously in the first few weeks after fertilization. Some of these chemical losses (also called "chemical pregnancies," [121]) are due to problems with the oocyte, but considering that 99% of sperm in the ejaculate die within a few minutes, and that two-thirds or even three-fourths of pregnancies terminate spontaneously argues against the existence of any kind of physiological sperm-selection mechanism.

On the other hand, there is some evidence that the granulosa cells surrounding the oocyte release progesterone and other chemotactic factors that attract sperm. To reach the surface of the egg (oolemma) and to fertilize it, the sperm must penetrate the corona radiata, and then the zona pellucida, as already discussed above. Several consecutive reactions must occur for this to happen.

The first is called "capacitation" [122] and, as the word suggests, means that sperm have to acquire the capacity to fertilize the egg. This became evident during the early days of *in vitro* fertilization, when the most direct approach – taking some sperm from a fresh ejaculate and putting them near the egg – proved unsuccessful. The sperm did not appear the least bit interested in fertilizing the egg, although they swarmed around it and were therefore clearly alive and motile.

Through observation and experimentation, it was found that there are lipid molecules such as cholesterol embedded in the membrane of a freshly ejaculated sperm head that prevent its ability to fertilize the egg. Once they were washed off by resuspension in fluid and centrifugation, the sperm readily penetrated the zona pellucida and fertilized the oocyte. We now know that lipid decapacitation factors [123] are secreted by the epididymal epithelium during the passage of sperm through the epididymis, a process that takes two to four weeks. Post-ejaculation, the fluid secretions of the cervix and uterus capacitate the sperm by washing off these lipid molecules, rendering sperm capable of fertilizing the oocyte. Once they become capacitated, sperm become hypermotile but have a limited life-span.

When the sperm encounter the oocyte–zona–granulosa complex, normally in the upper third of the fallopian tube (an area called the ampulla), the enzyme hyaluronidase on the sperm head dissolves hyaluronic acid, the "glue" that keeps granulosa cells together, allowing it to reach and bind to one of the proteins in the zona pellucida (ZP3). Three important reactions follow to ensure that fertilization by only one sperm occurs. The first, triggered by sperm binding to the zona pellucida, is the *acrosome reaction* [124]. The acrosomal cap dissolves, exposing and releasing proteases (e.g. acrosin) by exocytosis. This allows the spermatozoon to penetrate the glycoprotein matrix of the zona pellucida, which is only some 10–15 μm thick in humans. Once the sperm head contacts the oolemma, it binds to docking proteins, and this event produces a rapid depolarization of the oocyte membrane that begins at the point of contact and spreads throughout the cell, activating number of ionic and enzymatic second-messenger events within the oocyte that now recognizes that it has been fertilized.

This recognition triggers a second reaction, called the *cortical reaction* [125] in which thousands of small enzyme-containing vesicles floating just beneath the oolemma (in the cortex of the oocyte, hence, the name of the reaction) quickly migrate to the membrane, fuse with it, and dump their contents into the zona pellucida via an exocytotic process.

The cortical reaction thus initiates reaction 3: the *zona reaction* [126], in which the three principal proteins of the zona (ZP1, ZP2, and ZP3) first polymerize (ZP2 with ZP3) and are then cross-linked (by ZP1), thereby hardening the zona, so that it becomes more akin to an eggshell. In addition, in humans, a metalloproteinase called ovastacin is released from the cortical granules. By proteolytically cleaving the docking site on one of the zona proteins (ZP2), it prevents other sperm from binding and fertilizing the egg. This block to polyspermy [127] assures a diploid rather than a triploid zygote that would be created if two sperm fertilized one egg, creating three pronuclei and a zygote with 69 instead of 46 chromosomes.

Another less obvious biological challenge is the prevention of fertilization by gametes from different species. Species-specificity [128] has been recognized for some time, and appears to involve molecules present on both the sperm and the egg. The interaction of the acrosome-reacted head of the sperm with the zona of the egg can thus be viewed as an important recognition event that is a prerequisite for fertilization. At the same time, if the zona is chemically removed, cross-species fertilization [129] can indeed take place. Recognition of this fact led to a clinical test called the *hamster zona-free ovum test* (HZFO test, using hamster eggs and human sperm) that was once a part of the male infertility workup, although it has been replaced by newer diagnostics and is no longer used in the evaluation of infertility. Without the zona, the human sperm did fertilize the hamster egg (creating a "humster"), and the resulting zygote would undergo a few cell divisions before being terminated. The system is not perfect, e.g. some cross-fertilization has taken place to create hybrids such as mules, beefalo, ligers, zebroids, etc. Perhaps the most famous imaginary example is the centaur (half human, half horse), a creature featured in Greek mythology.

Once the penetrating sperm's DNA is endocytosed by the egg, it decondenses to form a male pronucleus. Meanwhile, the chromosomes of the secondary oocyte (which completed their first meiotic division during this month's menstrual cycle and entered the second meiotic division, pausing in metaphase of division 2, as already discussed in Chapter 2) rapidly complete their second meiotic division. The secondary oocyte is then briefly an ovum. Fusion of the male and female pronuclei then takes place, chromosomes intermingling to reinstate a complete 46 chromosome genome, creating a new diploid cell called the zygote (130).

As mentioned in Section 1.4 whether the baby will be male or female depends on the sex chromosome carried by the fertilizing sperm. If it is an X, the individual will be a female (XX); if Y, a genetic male (XY).

The zygote divides into two cells called blastomeres 16–30 hours postfertilization. Subsequent divisions increase the number of cells geometrically (2, 4, 8, 16, 32, etc.). Because the oocyte/zygote is so large, the first few divisions increase the number of cells while the volume of each cell is reduced and, after several days, forms a solid ball of smaller cells called the morula [131]. Still surrounded by the zona pellucida and some corona radiata cells, the morula is an undifferentiated structure in which each cell is like another. These totipotent stem cells are quite resilient, and if the morula divides into two parts (or even if a single cell breaks off of it), each can potentially grow into a complete individual.

3.2 Implantation

As the cells of the zygote divide and form the morula, the whole structure tumbles down the oviduct and passes into the cavity of the uterus five or six days after fertilization (Figure 3.1). Occasionally, it may attempt to implant somewhere within the fallopian tube, or, more rarely, tumble out of the oviduct into the abdominal cavity. This medically serious condition in which

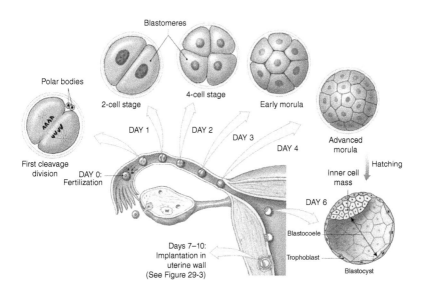

Blastomeres

Polar bodies

2-cell stage

4-cell stage

Early morula

First cleavage division

DAY 0: Fertilization

DAY 1

DAY 2

DAY 3

DAY 4

Advanced morula

Inner cell mass

Hatching

DAY 6

Blastocoele

Days 7–10: Implantation in uterine wall (See Figure 29-3)

Trophoblast

Blastocyst

Figure 3.1 Early embryology events.

a fertilized egg implants and grows outside of the main cavity of the uterus is called an ectopic pregnancy [132]. The tissues of the oviduct or abdomen cannot adapt properly in response to implantation and will ultimately be unable to accommodate the growing conceptus; left untreated, this condition becomes increasingly painful and can lead to rupture and internal bleeding.

Four or five days after fertilization, the morula becomes the blastocyst [133]. Specifically, the solid ball of cells in which every cell is exactly like another develops a fluid-filled center with an eccentric cell mass called the embryoblast (or inner cell mass) tucked within a surrounding sphere of trophoblast cells. The trophoblast cells, in turn, differentiate into cyto- and syncitio-trophoblasts and eventually form the placenta, while the inner cell mass becomes the embryo and differentiates into the endoderm, ectoderm, and mesoderm. Unlike the totipotent cells of the morula, the cells of the blastocyst are pluripotent stem cells, and – under the proper conditions – can be induced to differentiate into a variety of cell types, but cannot develop into a complete individual.

The blastocyst remains enclosed within the hardened zona pellucida until the time of implantation, which occurs approximately six days after fertilization. During the day or two that the blastocyst wanders around the uterus, seeking a favorable place to implant, it is nourished by the constituents of uterine fluid, which is largely derived from the stimulatory action of progesterone on the secretory activity of the endometrial glands.

At this time, the outer trophoblastic cells (syncitiotrophoblast) begin to secrete a hormone called human chorionic gonadotropin (hCG) [134] which is a glycoprotein that is very similar to the maternal luteinizing hormone (LH) we considered in light of the menstrual cycle.

The function of hCG is to rescue the corpus luteum (CL) in the ovary. The CL, in turn, secretes estrogen (E) and progesterone (P), sex steroids that maintain the integrity of the uterine endometrium. If pregnancy does not occur, the CL dies after about two weeks, and the resulting fall in E and P leads endometrial loss (menstruation). Since menstruation is incompatible with pregnancy, hCG secretion is a critical event because it assures the continued production of E and P by the CL. The amount of hCG in the circulation doubles every 48 hours, and peaks around 8–10 weeks of gestation. This exponential rise in hCG is vital, and a less-than-exponential rise may indicate that the pregnancy is failing (or possibly ectopic).

By week 8 postfertilization (week 10 of pregnancy, since human pregnancy is normally dated not from the day of ovulation and fertilization, but from the last menstrual period – LMP), the developing placenta is producing its own E and P in sufficient amounts to no longer require ovarian production, and becomes the primary site of sex steroid production. This event is called the luteo-placental shift [135], and is characterized by a peak in circulating hCG concentrations followed by gradual reduction. The amounts of E and P produced by the placenta quickly outpace the amount secreted by the CL, but some hCG is still made, and the CL remains viable and continues to secrete E and P throughout pregnancy, although its contribution is increasingly minor compared to that produced by the placenta.

The process of implantation coincides with endometrial decidualization [136]. Stimulated by progesterone, decidualization involves cellular hypertrophy, leading to large, loose, and sometimes multinucleated cells that contain significant amounts of glycogen and lipid. As the blastocyst begins to implant, it hatches from the zona pellucida, and – via the action of trophoblastic cells – initiates a decidual reaction. This leads to vasodilation of small endometrial vessels, increased capillary permeability and edema, and additional cellular proliferation within the decidua.

3.3 Multiple Births

Fraternal or dizygotic twins [137] occur when a woman ovulates two ova in one cycle, and both are fertilized. In this case, the two individuals may be of the same, or different sex, and are genetically no more similar than other any two siblings, except that they will be of the same age. Identical or monozygotic twins [138] occur either when the morula breaks apart into two parts, or if the inner cell mass separates into two parts during the blastocyst stage. The pattern of placentation is telling in this regard: a divided morula will differentiate into two blastocysts, and each individual will have their own placenta. On the other hand, if the inner cell mass divides within the blastocyst, the two individuals will share one placenta. In either case, the individuals will be genetically identical, and are therefore always of the same sex.

The incidence of twinning [139] is approximately 1/100 births. Fraternal twins are approximately twice as common as identical twins. Triplets occur at a frequency of $(0.01)^2$, or 1/10 000 births, quadruplets at $(0.01)^4$, or 1/1 000 000 births, etc. This frequency applies to natural pregnancies, of course, since several embryos may be transferred into the uterus during *in vitro* fertilization depending on the age and the health of the woman (normally a maximum of 4 for women of advanced reproductive age). Techniques have improved to the point where some clinics will only transfer one embryo into a healthy younger woman; in the case where multiple embryos implant successfully, a woman may undergo multifetal reduction, a surgical procedure that ablates all but one implantation. This procedure is normally performed during the first trimester, before week 12 of pregnancy.

3.4 Placentation

Proper development of the placenta is essential for successful pregnancy outcome, and the placenta initially dwarfs the embryo and early fetus, growing rapidly and differentiating into a functional structure. The functional units of a human placenta, which is hemochorial, are the fetal villi. The fetal villi begin to form on days 11–12 post-fertilization, extending into the small maternal lacunae that are created from endometrial blood vessels immediately after implantation. By the fourth week, the villi cover the entire surface of the chorionic sac. As the placenta matures, it becomes more eccentric (one-sided, relative to the fetus), and is eventually discoid in shape and quite substantial. At term (40 weeks), the human placenta may weigh a pound or more (Figure 3.2).

The term hemochorial is a clue to how it works. As the name suggests, hemo (= maternal blood) + chorial (fetal chorion) implies that maternal blood washes over the fetal villi, providing nutrition and carrying away waste. As the placenta develops, it becomes a chamber with a floor (the basal plate) and a roof (the chorionic plate). The space within the chamber is filled with a million or more fetal villi, which are small finger- or root-like structures that dangle from the chorionic plate and are arranged in areas called cotyledons. To continue the analogy of rootlets, instead of being filled with earth, however, the space between the villi (appropriately termed the intervillous space, or IVS) is filled with maternal blood that enters the placenta through maternal vessels called spiral arteries [140].

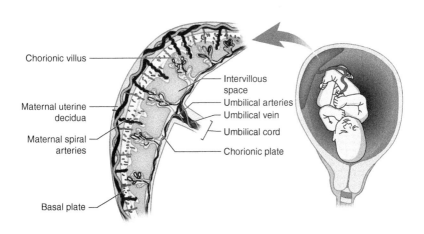

Chorionic villus

Maternal uterine decidua

Maternal spiral arteries

Basal plate

Intervillous space
Umbilical arteries
Umbilical vein
Umbilical cord
Chorionic plate

Figure 3.2 Structure of the human placenta.

This is a remarkable process that involves fetal trophoblastic cells literally crawling into the lumen of the small muscular spiral arteries in the endometrium through a process of *endovascular invasion*. By ablating the cells of the vascular wall (endothelium and vascular smooth muscle), the small vessels are remodeled into trumpet-shaped tubes that widen as they approach the basal plate and provide minimal resistance to blood flow, assuring vigorous perfusion of the IVS. Normally, there are some 20–50 spiral arteries that might be tapped to provide the maternal blood inflow into the IVS. The maternal blood washes over the villi and leaves the placenta via venules that eventually come together into veins, and drain into the inferior vena cava. Abrogation of this process (a situation in which the invasion is too shallow, not widening the vessels enough) is associated with preeclampsia, a form of hypertension that develops during pregnancy and that sometimes can lead to an extremely serious, even lethal condition of very high blood pressure and seizures called eclampsia.

The key to figuring out how the placenta functions lies in understanding the structure of a fetal villus [141]. Each villus consists of a shell (trophoblast cells) and an interior. The interior is a capillary loop that carries fetal blood into, and then back out of a villus. If you look at a villous in cross section, you would see two circular structures (the endothelium of the descending and ascending capillary) within a larger circular structure (the trophoblastic shell) that surrounds the capillaries.

A variety of molecules can pass from mother to fetus (and vice versa) via placental transport pathways [142] that are similar to those used by the gut: simple diffusion, facilitated diffusion (concentration-gradient driven but carrier-mediated), and energy-requiring active transport.

Oxygen diffuses from maternal blood to the fetal blood down a concentration gradient, and its effectiveness is enhanced by fetal hemoglobin, which has a higher affinity for oxygen than adult (maternal) hemoglobin. Conversely, wastes such as CO_2 diffuse from the fetal blood to the maternal blood.

Glucose, the molecular fuel for a growing fetus, passes across the placenta via facilitated diffusion. There are carrier molecules that shuttle glucose across the trophoblast cell, so the process is limited by the number of carrier molecules, and determined most directly by the concentration gradient. Gestational diabetes (GD, [143]) – a Type II diabetes that is characterized by elevated maternal insulin resistance, rather than a deficiency of insulin as in Type I – provides a good example of how physiological mechanisms can sometimes contribute to a pathological state. Because maternal cells are resistant to the action of insulin (which normally removes glucose from the blood by shuttling it into cells), higher-than-normal levels of glucose persist in the circulation following ingestion of a carbohydrate-rich meal. This increases the concentration gradient between the maternal blood in the IVS and the fetal blood within the villus. Since the process of facilitated diffusion is concentration-dependent, an excessive amount of glucose passes into the fetal blood. Particularly in the third trimester, this leads to a fetus growing too quickly and failing to mature as it should in the last few weeks of gestation. Thus, if untreated, GD babies are both overgrown and functionally immature. Treatment consists of normalizing the mother's glucose by diet and exercise, and requires the patient measuring her glucose several times a day, i.e. patient compliance. The effectiveness of treatment is therefore ultimately determined by the interaction between the physician's ability to communicate effectively, and the patient's own perceptions and character that determine compliance. In most hospitals in the United States, patients are screened for GD by an oral glucose tolerance test at 28 weeks of gestation.

Other substances, amino acids for example, pass across the placenta by active transport. Large, polar molecules (e.g. mother's insulin) tend not to cross the placenta, while small lipid-soluble molecules (e.g. mother's cholesterol) diffuse across quite easily. The trophoblast cells making up the shell of the villus are the primary gate-keepers in this regard, as once a molecule traverses across the trophoblast cell, it will readily enter the fetal capillary. Any recreational drug that produces a high (and therefore clearly passes the blood–brain barrier), will also easily traverse the placenta, since it is a much less selective barrier. Thus, if the mom has a glass of whiskey, or snorts some cocaine, the drug will pass to her baby, who is in a decidedly more vulnerable physiologic state because it is undergoing a high degree of cell division and differentiation. These processes are always subject to error, and the addition of a toxin such as alcohol, even in small quantities, carries increased risk of developmental damage. Similarly, if the mother takes antidepressants, or any other drug that has CNS actions, the baby will be subjected to their pharmacologic actions as well.

The passage of bacteria and viruses across the placenta is more complex, and precludes generalization. For example, a retrovirus like HIV does not pass across the placenta, but the baby can be infected during the process of birth through contact with maternal blood.

The fetal circulation [144] involves blood leaving the placenta by traveling from the capillaries in the villi, into small venules, and veins in the chorionic plate. The veins eventually converge to form one large vein (umbilical vein) that carries the blood within a structure called the umbilical cord into the body of the fetus.

Conversely, fetal arterial blood passes into two vessels called umbilical arteries that normally originate from the hypogastric arteries, which branch from the femoral arteries. Since we are bipedal, and have two legs (and two femoral arteries), two umbilical arteries return the blood to the placenta. These vessels are also ensheathed in the umbilical cord, thus, a cross section of the cord would reveal one umbilical vein and two umbilical arteries.

Although there is sometimes some confusion about the nomenclature, it makes perfect sense if you reason it out. Arteries carry blood away from the heart, and the umbilical arteries carry blood to the placenta. Veins return blood to the heart and, in this case, the fetal blood is transported via the umbilical vein, which enters through the umbilicus (future belly button) and leads to the fetal liver. Some flows through the liver, but about one-third flows around the liver in a bypass vessel called the ductus venosus. Either way, the venous blood eventually enters the inferior vena cava and flows into the right side of the fetal heart. The only difference is that oxygen concentrations are higher in the umbilical vein than in the umbilical arteries since – in the absence of air and functioning lungs – the placenta acts as the fetal lung by oxygenating the fetal blood within the villi with oxygen derived from the maternal arterial blood in the IVS.

3.5 The Endocrinology of Pregnancy

In addition to being the organ of nutrient and gaseous exchange, the placenta is also an important and versatile endocrine gland [145]. As noted above, the trophoblast cells produce hCG early on, and produce increasing amounts of estrogen and progesterone throughout pregnancy. It also secretes a plethora of other hormones, including human placental lactogen (hPL), hypothalamic-like hormones (GnRH, CRH, TRH), and pituitary-like hormones (ACTH, growth hormones).

Relative to the complex endocrinology of the menstrual cycle, the endocrine profile of pregnancy is much simpler. As already considered above, during the first trimester, hCG is secreted in increasing amounts, and peaks at around week 10 of pregnancy. Estrogen and progesterone [146] are produced in increasing amounts by the placenta throughout pregnancy, rising to a peak just before term. The circulating concentrations of estrogen reach 200–250 pg/ml, while those of progesterone attain 100–200 ng/ml, shortly before term. These values dwarf the highest values obtained during the menstrual cycle, with estrogen concentrations increasing approximately 100-fold, and progesterone concentrations increasing some 10- to 15-fold above those normally measured during the menstrual cycle.

A few additional points deserve mention:

- In comparing sex steroid circulating levels, it is important to distinguish between measures of concentration vs. molarity, e.g. picograms (pg) vs. picoliters (pl) for estrogen, and nanograms (ng) vs. nanoliters (nl) for progesterone, since both are in common use.

- While placental trophoblast cells can manufacture progesterone *de novo*, placental estrogen is derived from fetal androgens, placental progesterone, or other steroid precursors.

- In addition to 17β-estradiol (E2), which is the dominant estrogen in nonpregnant women, significant amounts of two additional estrogens are produced during gestation: estrone (E1) and estriol (E3) [147], with the latter attaining concentrations that approach or exceed those of 17β-estradiol (E2). In terms of biological activity, however, E2 is most potent.

Progesterone and estrogen have many important functions during gestation. Estrogens increase the size of the uterus and augment uterine blood flow, are critical in the timing of implantation, induce the formation of progesterone (and, near term, oxytocin) receptors in the uterus, enhance fetal organ development, stimulate maternal hepatic protein synthesis, and increase the mass of breast and adipose tissues. Progesterone is essential for maintaining uterine quiescence, and for survival of the early embryo. It also suppresses maternal immunological responses to fetal antigens, serves as a precursor for steroid production by the fetal adrenal cells, and stimulates myometrial growth.

Risking oversimplification, a good phraseology to remember when thinking about the actions of these hormones on the uterus is: "exciting estrogen" vs. "peaceful progesterone" since the former tends to be excitatory in terms of its effects on cellular functions such as ciliary and secretory activity and contractility, while progesterone – the progestational steroid – induces myometrial quiescence.

3.6 Prenatal Testing for Fetal Aneuplody and Other Maternal and Fetal Conditions

When the maternal (egg) and paternal (sperm) chromosomes combine after fertilization, each gamete should have a complete and correct complement of chromosomes, a condition termed euploidy. Occasionally, however, a pair of chromosomes fails to separate during the meiosis (nondisjunction, [148]). Following nondisjunction, which can occur during meiosis 1 (due to a failure of a pair of homologous chromosomes to separate) or in meiosis 2 (a failure of sister chromatids to separate), one of the daughter cells will have an extra copy of a chromosome, while the other will lack a chromosome. When the gametes combine during fertilization, a trisomy or a monosomy, respectively, will occur, resulting in an abnormal number of chromosomes (aneuploidy).

Monosomies are usually lethal, and the only survivors are those with a single X chromosome (Turner syndrome, [149]). These individuals are female and often have some gonadal dysgenesis. They are usually but not always infertile, of shorter stature, and have an increased frequency of congenital abnormalities.

Trisomy of the sex chromosomes can involve an extra copy of either the X chromosome (XXX = female, usually normal; XXY = Klinefelter syndrome [150]: infertile males, impaired intelligence, hypogonadal with low testosterone levels) or Y chromosome (XYY = males, often sterile, taller than average with some degree of mental impairment). Trisomy or monosomy can also occur in other chromosomes (autosomes). Individuals with Down syndrome, a trisomy of chromosome 21, will develop with mild-to-moderate intellectual disability, short stature, and a characteristic facial appearance. Its overall incidence is 1 in 700 pregnancies, but the likelihood of having a child with Down syndrome increases with maternal age, and is usually tested for in women older than 35.

As the placenta develops, the fetus becomes surrounded by two concentric spherical membranous layers. From outside in, these fetal membranes [151] are the chorion and the amnion, and the inner space in which the fetus floats is filled with amniotic fluid. Amniocentesis [152], first used in 1956, entails using an ultrasound probe to visualize the position of the fetus, inserting a needle transabdominally, and drawing out 10–20 ml of amniotic fluid. The fetal cells floating within the amniotic fluid can be centrifuged and analyzed for aneuploidy by performing a chromosomal smear. Because the procedure is invasive and requires a substantial volume of fluid, it should not be used until after week 14 of gestation.

Chorionic villous sampling (CVS, [153]) is a more recent technique (first described in 1983) that involves passing a catheter through the cervix and into the uterus to collect a snippet of placental tissue containing chorionic villi. Since the placenta is a fetal organ, the biopsied cells can be dissociated and subjected to chromosomal analysis. The major advantage of CVS is that it can be performed earlier than amniocentesis (after week 10), making elective abortion a less complicated procedure. On the other hand, some studies have found an elevated rate of birth defects in children of mothers that have undergone CVS, and an increased risk of miscarriage and infection.

There is always a small amount of fetal DNA in the maternal circulation, and the sensitivity of molecular techniques has improved enough in the last two decades to allow the isolation of cell-free fetal DNA [154] from a sample of maternal plasma. Commercial kits for detecting not just aneuploidy (e.g. trisomy of chromosomes 13, 18, and 21), but also paternity, sex, and congenital adrenal hyperplasia are now available and in increasingly wide use in view of their only requiring a simple blood draw.

Analyses of maternal blood (rather than fetal DNA) have been used for many years for obstetric diagnostic purposes. We have already considered hCG, for example, the basis of the early pregnancy test, and maternal serum alpha-fetoprotein (AFP) is useful for detecting neural tube defects such as spina bifida. Although much research effort has been put into developing biomarkers that predict gestational disease such as preeclampsia, at this time, their utility is limited.

3.7 Maternal Adaptations During Pregnancy

The secretion of hCG begins within a week of fertilization at the embryonic blastocyst stage. At this point, the conceptus is so small that it would not be visible to the naked eye without intense scrutiny, yet it is already watching out for its own survival. This remarkable avarice of new life cannot be overstated. In fact, in addition to hCG, the zygote secretes many other molecules – collectively termed early pregnancy proteins [155] – which are absorbed into the maternal systemic circulation, and that begin to induce a range of adaptive changes in the maternal organism.

This molecular signaling is all the zygote has to work with, since there are no nerves running from the embryo or fetus to the mother, leaving soluble signaling as the only option. The net effect is to induce a variety of changes in the maternal cardiovascular, respiratory, and reproductive systems. There are also changes in the immune system, in the chemistry and composition of the blood, in metabolism, and in CNS and GI function.

The cardiovascular system [156] undergoes three major changes: (i) the work of the heart is substantially increased, as evidenced by a 15–20% increase in heart rate (pulse increases by about 15 beats/min) as well as stroke volume (+15%), increasing cardiac output by >30%. This increase in contractility is often accompanied by the development of what are termed physiologic murmurs, since systolic murmurs are present in 80%, and diastolic murmurs in 20% of pregnancies.

At the same time, (ii) the plasma volume increases substantially, largely through an activation of the plasma renin–angiotensin system that leads to elevated aldosterone secretion and the reabsorption of sodium and water by the kidneys. Normal plasma volume expansion is on the order of 40% (this is for a singleton pregnancy; a woman carrying twins or triplets may expand her plasma volume by 60% or more). In a nonpregnant woman, the combination of increased cardiac output and plasma volume would increase blood pressure significantly.

Keep in mind that the equation for mean arterial pressure – *cardiac output × total peripheral* resistance – does not even take plasma volume into account. Clearly, adding fluid to a closed system will increase pressure unless the volume of the system can expand, or if new vascular growth occurs. During pregnancy, the body utilizes both adaptations to its advantage by creating a new vascular organ (the placenta) and by peripheral vasodilation, particularly of the smaller arteries and arterioles that are the primary site of peripheral resistance.

As a result, (iii) systemic blood pressure does not normally increase; in fact, it often decreases during early and midpregnancy, and returns to its normal level by term, following a U-shaped curve. The three major cardiovascular adaptations are therefore increased cardiac output, increased plasma volume, and decreased peripheral resistance (due to vasodilation and growth of new uterine vessels). These cardiovascular adaptations are already detectable by week seven of pregnancy, when the fetus is only the size of a blueberry, attesting to its ability to signal and induce major adaptive changes in the maternal organism.

On the respiratory side [157], the mother must breathe for two, and minute ventilation increases accordingly as pregnancy progresses. Tidal volume increases during pregnancy, and dyspnea (a sense of breathing discomfort) is a common complaint in the third trimester. One mechanism for inducing hyperventilation is a central action of progesterone on the respiratory center in the medulla, an effect that is also detectable in nonpregnant women during the luteal vs. follicular phase of the menstrual cycle, when progesterone levels are highest.

The uterus [158] is a small muscular organ in the nonpregnant state, weighing about 40 g. During pregnancy, it increases approximately 25× in mass, such that uterine weight (this does not include the fetoplacental contents) at term may approach or exceed 1200 g. The increase in myometrial muscle mass is essential for producing the forceful contractions required for parturition. In the six weeks after birth (called the puerperium), the uterus shrinks to almost its nonpregnant size (50–70 g). The increase in size is due to a combination of hyperplasia and hypertrophy; following some initial hyperplasia, as pregnancy progresses, each smooth muscle cell increases substantially in length and width due to increased protein synthesis and actin–myosin content.

3.8 Embryonic and Fetal Growth

The embryonic period [159] is defined as the first seven weeks post-fertilization (nine weeks of pregnancy using conventional LMP dating). All of the major organ systems are created during this period, even though at the end of embryonic life, the fetus may only weigh 1 or 2 g.

The fetal period [160] spans the remainder of pregnancy: 9–40 weeks post-fertilization, although it would be much shorter if a baby is born prematurely. The age at which a child can be born and survive (albeit with intensive medical support) is currently 23–24 weeks of gestation. A 22-week-old fetus weighs only a pound, and has less than a 10% chance of survival. He or she will also manifest with a host of medical problems including neurological defects, and require respiratory support. Even a few weeks make a big difference in this regard; by 27 or 28 weeks, >75% of premature babies will survive (2016 data).

3.9 Labor and Parturition

The uterus is normally quiescent during pregnancy, although many women feel occasional uncoordinated contractions as term approaches (Braxton Hicks contractions). The reason for the quiescence is largely due to the actions of progesterone (progesterone block, [161]), which inhibits smooth muscle contractility via several different mechanisms, including hyperpolarization of the smooth muscle membrane (preventing calcium entry) and regulating genetic expression. An example of the latter might be an inhibitory effect on the expression of receptors that mediate vasoconstriction in response to endogenous vasoactive molecules (e.g. oxytocin, thromboxane).

As term approaches, a complex interplay of fetal, maternal, and mechanical factors leads to the initiation of coordinated, rhythmic contractions called labor [162]. First, the growing conceptus imposes a stretch on the uterine smooth muscle, increasing the wall tension. Smooth muscle stretch increases excitability by inducing depolarization and calcium entry.

Second, the ratio of progesterone to estrogen decreases. While this event is quite prominent in many animals, in humans, total progesterone concentrations do not decrease. Rather, its effective concentration may be reduced by a rise in binding proteins, or a decline in the number of myometrial receptors.

Third, myometrial, decidual, and chorionic prostaglandin production (especially that of $PGF_{2\alpha}$ and PGE_2, both potent constrictors of smooth muscle) is increased, stimulating the onset of labor. For this reason, aspirin or ibuprofen (which inhibits cyclooxygenase, the enzyme that forms prostaglandins from arachidonic acid) is contraindicated in late pregnancy.

Fourth, myometrial sensitivity to oxytocin is increased due to an upregulation of oxytocin receptors and an increase in circulating levels of oxytocin. This potent vasoconstrictor is produced by the pituitary of the mother and of the fetus, and a synthetic analogue (Pitocin) is sometimes given to induce labor.

Two final considerations. First, keep in mind that the contractions of the uterus must be coordinated in terms of not only force, but frequency and spatial pattern. Contractions that start at the cervix and proceed to the fundus (top part) of the uterus would hardly be helpful. Second, an underlying question we have not addressed is whether labor is initiated by the mother or fetus [163]. The best answer is probably "both," although recent studies suggest that the fetus may play the dominant role, and most evidence points to the maturation and activation of the fetal corticotropin-releasing hormone (CRH)/adrenocorticotropin hormone (ACTH)/cortisol axis, which then alters placental signaling mechanisms, e.g. production of sex steroids and oxytocin.

Labor is divided into three phases [164]. The first stage is by far the longest and most painful. As contractions increase in regularity, force, and frequency, the cervix (which has been softened, or "ripened" by the actions of pregnancy hormones) begins to dilate, and so the first stage of labor is called the *dilatation stage*. It is often preceded by, or coincident with the rupture of the amniotic sac ("breaking of the waters"), and the process of cervical maturation involves both dilation and a process of shortening and thinning called cervical effacement. This stage can last >24 hours and is further divided into three phases: early labor (which begins with the onset of labor until the cervix has dilated to 3 cm), active labor (cervical effacement and dilation to 7 cm), and the transition phase (7 cm to full dilation).

Once the cervix has dilated and effaced sufficiently to permit the passage of the head of the fetus (normally 9–10 cm), the second stage of labor (*expulsion phase*) begins. This is where the mother bears down, trying to push the baby out, and lasts anywhere from a few minutes to just over an hour. The third phase of labor is that of *placental delivery*, which begins when the baby is born and continues until the placenta is expelled. It can be of variable length, generally from 15 minutes to 1 hour. Once a woman has had a child, the process of labor in subsequent pregnancies is usually less painful, and the dilation and expulsion phases are shorter.

The process of birth is traumatic for the baby, and requires a number of rapid adaptations, including the vasodilation of the pulmonary tree and the first breath, a shutting down of blood flow to the placenta (as it is no longer performing any useful function), and the rapid induction of cardiovascular adaptations required for normal life. These changes are preceded by several weeks of more subtle preparation, e.g. changes in the immune system, metabolic and liver function, and production of surfactant in the lungs.

The World Health Organization (WHO) defines preterm delivery [165] as delivery before 37 weeks of gestation (35 weeks post-fertilization) and premature birth may occur spontaneously, or be medically induced (e.g. in severe cases of preeclampsia). Management involves the administration of glucocorticoids to accelerate lung maturation, and surgical delivery via caesarean section.

3.10 Lactation and Breastfeeding

The newborn must be provided with oral nutrients, and be able to excrete wastes via the kidney and GI tract, as he or she now lack the placental interface for carrying out the respiratory, nutritive, and excretory functions.

In mammals, the feeding of the young is accomplished by lactation – maternal production and secretion of milk [166]. The body begins to prepare for milk production early in pregnancy, in fact, many women report enlargement (and, sometimes, tenderness) of the breasts as one of the first signs of pregnancy.

The adult breast consists of a cluster of 15–25 lactiferous ducts that converge upon the nipple. During pregnancy, the hormones progesterone, prolactin, and placental lactogen (hPL) play a dominant role in stimulating the growth of the breasts, particularly development of the tubuloalveolar secretory units and ducts.

During pregnancy, the high concentrations of progesterone and estrogen inhibit actual milk production, which would be counterproductive prior to parturition. Once a child is born, the E and P levels decrease precipitously, and this block is removed. In addition to the aforementioned hormones, growth and remodeling of the breasts and the production of milk require the actions of a number of other hormones that exert a cooperative or permissive influence. These include glucocorticoids, insulin, and the thyroid hormone thyroxine. The process of breast growth includes proliferation and branching of the lactiferous ducts, enlargement of the alveolar units, and accumulation of adipose and connective tissue.

The production and secretion of milk is accomplished by alveolar epithelial cells [167] that absorb nutrients from the bloodstream and synthesize the various nutrient components of milk, including proteins, lipids, and carbohydrates. These cells are quite active metabolically, and possess a large amount of rough endoplasmic reticulum that is involved in protein synthesis. Toward the end of pregnancy, the number of Ig-A-secreting lymphocytes increases, as does their secretory activity. As a result, the Ig-A crosses the epithelial cell via transcytosis and is deposited into the lumen, which is filled with milk. This is an important mechanism for providing the newborn with immediate passive immunity. The first milk, called colostrum [168], is a particularly rich and complex mixture of nutrients, and contains these maternal antibodies that help prime the newborn's immune system.

Although the production of milk involves the coordinated action of a number of hormones, as the name implies, prolactin secreted by the anterior pituitary is foremost among them. Lactating women may produce up to 600 ml of milk initially, and as much as a liter or more by the sixth postpartum month. Its composition changes over time, with highest levels of protein initially, followed by a progressive decrease, while the content of lipid, lactose, and water-soluble vitamins increases. For this reason, the appearance of milk changes from yellowish colostrum to whiter and less viscous as a woman continues to lactate.

The process of secreting milk is called milk let-down [169], and the mechanism is a neuroendocrine arc that involves the suckling reflex. Unlike most reflexes that have neural afferent and efferent arcs, the afferent arc of the suckling reflex is neural, while the efferent arc is neuroendocrine.

Sensory receptors in the nipple initiate nerve impulses that reach the hypothalamus via ascending fibers in the spinal cord and then via the mesencephalon. These fibers terminate in the supraoptic and paraventricular nuclei in the hypothalamus.

The efferent arc consists of nerve fibers that descend from the hypothalamus into the posterior pituitary (also called the neurohypophysis) from which they release oxytocin. The oxytocin travels via the bloodstream, and binds to receptors on myoepithelial cells, spindle-shaped muscle cells that wrap around each alveolus. When they constrict, the intra-alveolar pressure increases, forcing milk into the main collecting ducts. The milk let-down reflex can be conditioned so that the sound of a baby crying, or even the mother's awareness that it is time to feed the child, will induce oxytocin secretion.

Prolactin [170] levels increase progressively during pregnancy, but begin to decline shortly after parturition, reaching near pregestation levels by five or six months. Suckling, however, elicits a rapid and significant rise in plasma prolactin, with the exact amount being dependent on the intensity and duration of nipple stimulation. In this way, a system is set up for producing milk based on demand. If a woman decides to stop breast feeding, some swelling of the breasts occurs, leading to an increase in local pressure at the alveolar level, resulting in vascular stasis and alveolar regression.

One side effect of high prolactin levels is a contraceptive effect achieved by the inhibition of GnRH. The contraceptive influence is moderate, particularly when breast feeding is supplemented by bottle feeding. In women who choose not to breast feed, the menstrual cycle may return within a month or two of delivery, while lactating women undergo a period of several months of lactational amenorrhea. Once cycles return, the first few may be anovulatory, with normal cyclicity and ovulation returning thereafter.

A growing body of research evidence suggests that breastfeeding provides a number of beneficial effects to both mother and child [171]. For the mother, these include the promotion of uterine involution after birth, a reduction in the risk or postpartum hemorrhage, as well as lowering the risk of developing ovarian and breast cancer, and an enhancement of bonding to the child.

For the infant, the immuno-protective benefits of colostrum have already been discussed above. In addition, children who are breastfed have a reduced incidence of ear infections, pneumonia, enterocolitis, and gastroenteritis. They also have a smaller chance of sudden infant death syndrome (SIDS) and may experience long-term benefits such as a reduced likelihood of developing diabetes later in life, and potentially improved cognition.

3.11 Long-Term Health Effects of Pregnancy on Mother and Child

During its time *in utero*, the fetus is subject to a constantly changing maternal endocrine milieu and, indirectly, to external (environmental, medical) influences that affect maternal physiology. This is a burgeoning field of research called the developmental origins of health and disease (DOHaD, [172]) that is yielding some interesting insights. For example, maternal anxiety and stress (or, more accurately distress) can lead to the development of higher blood pressures in her offspring, likely due to elevated maternal cortisol being transferred to the fetus. Similarly, maternal hyperthyroidism has potential consequences for fetal neurological development and may predispose to hypertension, as well as a greater likelihood of the child developing psychological problems later in life. And it is well known that exposure to toxins and/or medicines may imprint upon the physiology of her offspring with medical or psychological consequences, with fetal alcohol syndrome (FAS) being the most well-recognized example. Since understanding fetal programming of the adult in the human requires decades, most DOHaD studies to date have been carried out in animals with short life spans, most commonly rodents. For this reason, the situation in humans is less clear, although several lines of parallel and confirmatory evidence are emerging. In fact, the original impetus for the fetal origins of adult disease was based on the concept put forth by Dr. David Barker (termed the "Barker Hypothesis") which was, in turn, predicated on the study of offspring of women who experienced malnutrition during the Dutch famine imposed by the Germans during the Second World War.

Pregnancy also leaves an indelible mark on the maternal organism. For example, women with pregnancies complicated by preeclampsia are more likely to develop hypertension and cardiovascular disease later in life, and gestational diabetics have a 3–4× increased chance of developing Type 2 diabetes as they age. What is not known is whether this is truly a consequence of the diseased pregnancy, or if the mother's phenotype was already compromised and in a presymptomatic phase, but that the stress of pregnancy became manifest in her developing gestational disease. Additional studies are needed to settle this question of consequence vs. predisposition [173].

4

The Human Sexual Response

The physiological response of the human body to sexual stimulation is most often divided into five phases that are based on the classification scheme proposed by Masters and Johnson [174] – desire, excitement, plateau, orgasm, and resolution. Although these phases are somewhat arbitrary, as sexual arousal is a continuum, it does allow us to separate and study the components of the human sexual response with greater ease.

4.1 Desire Phase

The sexiest part of our bodies is – without a doubt – the brain. It is the home of the libido and the "organ of desire." This is evident through the maelstrom of feelings we experience when attracted to another person in a physical way, and the wonderful way that attraction and romance can color and permeate everyday reality.

The limbic system [175] of the brain mediates many of our emotional and sexual feelings, although it itself is subject to modulation by a variety of sensory and hormonal inputs. For example, something as fleeting as a dream may change one's feelings for another person, and leave an intense impression that fades over the next day or two. At the same time, one must

Physiology of Human Reproduction: Notes for Students,
First Edition. George Osol.
© 2021 John Wiley & Sons Ltd. Published 2021 by John Wiley & Sons Ltd.

wonder whence the dream came from, and whether it was the dream that woke the desire, or the desire that created the dream. Each person has their own level of desire, or libido [176] that can be modulated by circumstance, state of health, state of life, and perhaps even diet. Libido is a complicated but fascinating area of psychobiology for which there are few concrete correlates. In general, androgens are associated with (but by no means solely responsible for) libido in both men and women. Women who have excess androgens (in some disease states, for example, like polycystic ovarian syndrome) may experience an elevated sex drive, with adrenal dehydroepiandrosterone (DHEA) being most directly implicated. Women who seek help for reduced sex drive may be prescribed low-dose androgens; similarly, in men, castration or medicines that alter androgen metabolism may reduce sex drive.

4.2 Excitement Phase

The excitement phase can be stimulated by a memory, an odor, or something visual (we are a very visual species in terms of attraction), or it can be physical – a touch, a caress, a kiss.

Arousal in the male leads to penile erection due to the inflow of blood into the three cylinder-shaped bundles of erectile tissue (one corpus spongiosum and two corpora cavernosa) in the penis via the parasympathetic-nitric oxide mechanism discussed in Section 1.7, causing it to fill, swell, and become rigid (tumescent), and to stand away from the body. The scrotal sac is slightly raised due to its muscular contraction, drawing the testes upward.

During sexual arousal in the female [177], the vestibular glands and the walls of the vagina begin to secrete a lubricating vaginal fluid. Increased permeability secondary to vasodilation of veins within the wall of the vagina leads to a transudation of fluid across the vaginal wall. There are also increased secretions from the cervix. The increased blood flow confers turgidity to the inner two-thirds of the vagina, which lengthens. The uterus rises in the pelvis, also secondary to increased blood flow. The labia majora (outer vaginal lips) open, and the labia minora (inner vaginal lips) thicken and become more turgid. The clitoris swells and lengthens, as its erectile tissues – located beneath the skin in two cords that surround the vaginal opening (vestibule) – become engorged with blood. The breasts respond to stimulation initially with erection of the nipples, and with an increase in mammary blood flow.

4.3 Plateau Phase

A number of general body reactions characterize the plateau phase in men and women. This is the time during which sexual arousal is elevated to the point where the individual may enter the orgasmic phase.

Blood flow to the skin is increased, producing a visible sex flush [178], usually first visible on the abdomen and spreading to the chest and breasts, face, and other parts of the body. Masters and Johnson found that 75% of the women they observed developed the sex flush on occasion. The plateau phase is also characterized by deeper breathing and an increase in heart rate. The outer third of the vagina swells as more blood flows into it secondary to parasympathetic stimulation and arterial relaxation. The swollen outer vagina and labia minora form a long elevation that is known as the orgasmic platform. The clitoris, erect and palpable, and retracts beneath the clitoral hood (secondary to swelling of the labia minora), but remains quite sensitive to direct stimulation.

In the man, the penis grows slightly larger and the head (glans) develops a reddish purple color and becomes shiny. During intense arousal, few drops of sticky watery fluid (mucus) appear from the opening at its tip (the meatus) and the testes are drawn still higher and closer to the body.

4.4 Orgasmic Phase

If sexual stimulation is appropriate – in women, especially in terms of clitoral stimulation (few women experience orgasm based on solely vaginal stimulation) – orgasm is initiated as the orgasmic platform [179] which contracts rhythmically 3–15 times at ~0.8 second intervals. The achievement of orgasm is a delicate interplay of physical stimulation and mental process – in both men and women, the psyche has to cooperate for orgasm to be achieved. Once orgasm actually begins, it continues as an involuntary reflex, with rhythmic contractions of the orgasmic platform, along with the other structures within the pelvis, giving a unique feeling of intense sexual pleasure. Female orgasm is associated with increased cervical and vaginal secretions and, unlike the male (who experiences a refractory period once he ejaculates – a period when he is unable to develop an erection and ejaculate), in the female, multiple orgasms can be experienced during a single sexual experience.

The question of whether women ejaculate has been considered for a long time; before the seventeenth century, the vaginal lubricant was assumed to be a female "ejaculate" analogous to male semen, and therefore essential for conception. Interestingly, this misunderstanding formed the basis of theological tolerance of female masturbation during coitus. The reasoning was based on the fact that, if a woman did not reach orgasm during coitus, it was permissible do to so by manipulation, otherwise, she would not be able to complement the male semen with her own to make conception possible.

In 1950, Ernest Gräfenberg published a paper in which he claimed that there was an erotic zone on the anterior wall of the vagina along the course of the urethra, where there is a thickening of the urethral tissue (called the urethral sponge). This area was subsequently called the "G Spot" [180] in his honor.

When properly stimulated, it leads to orgasm, and to the emission of fluid through the urethra that is similar to the male ejaculate in that it contains the enzyme prostatic-specific antigen (PSA), although this is something of a misnomer since females do not have a prostate gland. Subsequent studies have highlighted the association between this sensitive area that contains glandular tissue (e.g. Skene's glands, sometimes called the "female prostate") and sexual arousal and female ejaculation. There is some association between this anatomical area and elevated levels of phosphodiesterase-5 (PDE-5), an enzyme that breaks down cGMP and is the principal target of sildenafil (Viagra); in men, inhibition of PDE-5 facilitates erection since cGMP levels are increased, leading to penile vasodilation and a filling of the erectile tissues. In women, sildenafil can facilitate sexual arousal, most likely also through its ability to enhance genital blood flow.

4.5 Resolution Phase

The resolution phase is divided into two stages in the male. First, the penis shrinks to about half its fully erect size. In the second phase, the penis returns to its normal flaccid size from the semi-erect or rigid phase. The second stage takes longer than the first and, as the penis shrinks, the scrotum becomes loose, allowing the testes to descend away from the body. A feeling of sleepiness and mental and muscular relaxation follows.

In the female, both nerve traffic and blood flow to the genital area decrease, leading to a return of the clitoris and vagina to their normal color, size, and position over a period of about 15–20 minutes. Respiration and heart rate return to normal, and a period of peace and relaxation follows. Some women describe feeling sleepy, others feel alert or even exhilarated during the resolution phase.

Notably, sexual desire and sexual performance do not necessarily decline with age. In fact, some women experience a heightened sex drive after menopause that may be related to endocrinologic changes, but also to psychological factors, such as no longer having to worry about becoming pregnant. In men, sexual function can be maintained into old age, although everything may take a bit longer to accomplish, and some men in the eight or even ninth decade of life have fathered children with much younger women.

5   Age-Related Changes in the Reproductive System

5.1 Childhood and Adolescence

Once a child is born, the reproductive system remains quiescent until the time of puberty, which occurs around the age of 10–11 in girls and 11–12 in boys here in the United States. Puberty [181] is not an event, rather, it is a coordinated, multifaceted process that transforms the physiology of a child into that of a reproductive-capable adult. The changes are many, and "coming of age" involves much more than just maturation of the reproductive system. Anyone who has lived with a teenager, or remembers their teenage years objectively (!) knows that those years can be difficult, moody, and unpredictable (CNS effects). There are also changes in appearance, weight, growth rate, and intellectual capacity. While almost every organ in the body is affected, it is safe to say that the driving influence behind all these changes is the endocrine system or, more specifically, that portion of the endocrine system that regulates reproductive function and that we have discussed in earlier chapters on the adult male and nonpregnant female.

The hypothalamus is capable of interpreting and integrating many different stimuli and responding by producing small peptide molecules called releasing hormones that regulate anterior

Physiology of Human Reproduction: Notes for Students,
First Edition. George Osol.

pituitary function. Some of its axons also extend to and terminate in the posterior pituitary (neurohypophysis), where they release oxytocin, previously considered with respect to milk let-down. The hypothalamic–pituitary–gonadal axis undergoes prolonged and multiphasic activation *in utero* during the processes of sex determination and gonadal genesis. Once a child is born, he or she is deprived of maternal steroids passing across the placenta, and of the steroids derived from the placenta itself. This leads to a wave of activation (increased gonadotropins, estrogen, and testosterone) that crests at approximately 3 months of age, when levels are in the low-normal adult range. Circulating concentrations of the reproductive hormones then decline over the course of the next six months and remain low throughout childhood, maintaining reproductive quiescence.

During adult life, one would expect low steroid levels to stimulate the hypothalamus and pituitary, but the entire system is suppressed during childhood by a combination of mechanisms. These include inhibition of GnRH secretion by circulating steroids, as the hypothalamus is exquisitely sensitive to their feedback effect [182] during childhood. Interestingly, the system itself is responsive, i.e. injections of GnRH in the proper pattern would stimulate the onset of puberty, even in a very young child.

Although the molecular triggers that initiate pubertal development [183] are likely multiple, one system that has received increasing attention in the last decade is kisspeptin [184]. Loss-of-function mutations in the gene that encodes its cognate receptor (KISS1R) are associated with hypogonadotropic hypogonadism, while a genetic mutation that induces early activation of this receptor was identified in a girl with central precocious puberty.

Puberty is thought to be initiated by the activation of kisspeptin neurons in the arcuate nucleus of the hypothalamus. These project to, and are able to activate hypothalamic GnRH neurons, thereby initiating its pulsatile release, gonadotropin (LH, FSH) secretion, and subsequent sexual maturation. Kisspeptin, in turn, is regulated by other compounds, e.g. Neurokinin B [185], and other signaling systems have also been implicated in the initiation of puberty in humans. For example, childhood obesity is associated with early puberty onset, particularly in girls. Although the neural pathways are not well-defined, one mechanism that has received considerable attention is that of the adipose hormone leptin [186] playing a role in activating kisspeptin secretion which, in turn, stimulates GnRH pulsatility.

5.2 Puberty

In girls, the process of puberty [187] – a period during which fertility is acquired – begins with the appearance of breast buds (the process is called the *thelarche*), and the appearance of pubic hair. Axillary hair and an increased rate of growth follow within one to two years, and the first period (the menarche) marks the beginning of subsequent menstrual cyclicity. In the United States, the age of menarche now stands at just under 12 years.

In boys, the first sign of puberty is an enlargement of the testes, followed by the appearance of pubic hair and penile enlargement. On average, the peak spurt of growth, and development of axillary hair in boys occurs two years later than in girls. Late puberty in males is associated with a broadening of the shoulders and depending of the voice, and the appearance of facial hair.

5.3 The Aging Male and Female

Male sexual function declines gradually with age [188] with the incidence of erectile dysfunction increasing after the age of 40, and a gradual reduction in testosterone concentrations, sperm count, and sexual performance. Thus, while there may be some loss of fertility, the basic male reproductive functions are generally maintained well into old age, and some men in the eighth or even ninth decade of life have successfully fathered children. Libido may be maintained, or decrease, especially in response to infirmity and illness, and/or due to side effects of common medicines.

Prostatic enlargement [189] occurs with time in all men due to a slow process of benign prostatic hypertrophy (BPH) along with an increased incidence of prostate cancer. In either case, because the prostate is encapsulated in relatively inelastic connective tissue, benign or malignant hypertrophy of the prostatic stroma will lead to a compression of the urethra, difficulty in urination, and nocturia.

By the time a woman reaches the fifth decade or, in some cases, earlier, she may begin to experience menstrual cycles that are irregular. This phase is called the *climacteric period*, and may last several years, and terminate in the complete absence of menstrual periods (menopause, [190]).

Some women experience symptoms associated with estrogen withdrawal [191], including hot flashes, headache, sweating, and insomnia. With the loss of ovarian follicles, estrogen cannot be produced and its loss leads to a compensatory elevation in circulating gonadotropins. Thus, the hormonal life pattern is one of low estrogen and low gonadotropins during childhood, elevated gonadotropins and estrogens during the reproductive years, and low estrogen and high gonadotropins in the postmenopausal period; in fact, gonadotropins were first isolated from the urine of Italian nuns!

The same pattern is present in males, if one substitutes "testosterone" for "estrogen," although the decrease in testosterone levels and increase in gonadotropins is more gradual, lacking the more discrete nature of the climacteric period and menopause.

The loss of estrogen postmenopause leads to some atrophy of the reproductive organs, and an increased risk of developing osteoporosis and cardiovascular disease. As we already have discussed, sex steroids have effects on almost every organ, including the brain, and so loss of estrogen may be associated with some emotional and cognitive changes that are highly variable from individual to individual.

Some women have elected to have a child after menopause, which is possible with the administration of estrogen and progesterone. This demonstrates that, although ovarian function has ceased, the organs dependent on ovarian hormones can still respond when given the appropriate signals.

Appendix A Detailed Anatomy of the Male and Female Reproductive Systems

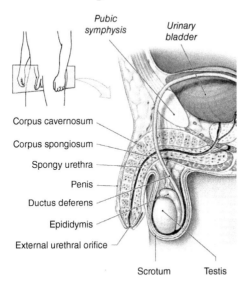

Figure A.1 Anatomy of the male reproductive system, saggital section.

Physiology of Human Reproduction: Notes for Students,
First Edition. George Osol.
© 2021 John Wiley & Sons Ltd. Published 2021 by John Wiley & Sons Ltd.

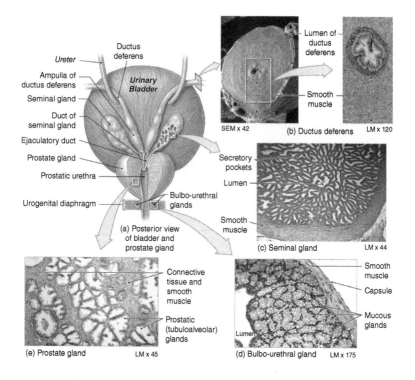

Figure A.2 Anatomy of the male reproductive system showing internal structures and histology.

Source: Parts (c) and (d), Frederic, H. M. et al. (2009), *The Reproductive System*, Pearson Education, Inc., publishing as Pearson Benjamin Cummings.

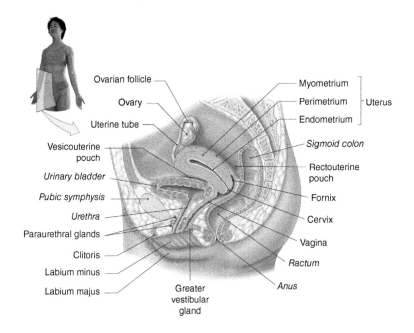

Ovarian follicle
Ovary
Uterine tube
Vesicouterine pouch
Urinary bladder
Pubic symphysis
Urethra
Paraurethral glands
Clitoris
Labium minus
Labium majus
Greater vestibular gland

Myometrium
Perimetrium ⎤ Uterus
Endometrium ⎦
Sigmoid colon
Rectouterine pouch
Fornix
Cervix
Vagina
Ractum
Anus

Figure A.3 Anatomy of the female reproductive system saggital section.

Source: Frederic, H. M. et al. (2009), *The Reproductive System*, Pearson Education,Inc., publishing as Pearson Benjamin Cummings.

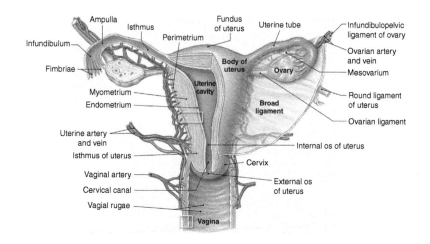

Figure A.4 Anatomy of the female reproductive system, showing internal structures.

Source: Frederic, H. M. et al. (2009), *The Reproductive System*, Pearson Education, Inc., publishing as Pearson Benjamin Cummings.

Index

Note: Page numbers in *italic* refer to figures.
Page numbers in **bold** refer to tables.

Physiology of Human Reproduction: Notes for Students,
First Edition. George Osol.
© 2021 John Wiley & Sons Ltd. Published 2021 by John Wiley & Sons Ltd.